THE HAND

EXAMINATION AND DIAGNOSIS

AMERICAN SOCIETY FOR SURGERY OF THE HAND

THIRD EDITION

CHURCHILL LIVINGSTONE
NEW YORK, EDINBURGH, LONDON, MELBOURNE

Library of Congress Cataloging-in-Publication Data

The Hand, examination and diagnosis / American Society for
  Surgery of the Hand. — 3rd ed.
    p.   cm.
    Includes bibliographical references.
    ISBN 0-443-08715-6
    1. Hand—Wounds and injuries—Diagnosis.   2. Hand—
Abnormalities—Diagnosis.   3. Hand—Diseases—Diagnosis.
4. Hand—Examination.   I. American Society for Surgery of the
Hand.
    [DNLM: 1. Hand—abnormalities.   2. Hand Deformities,
Acquired—diagnosis.   3. Hand Injuries—diagnosis.   WE 830
H2308]
RD559.H359   1990
617.5′75075—dc20
DNLM/DLC
for Library of Congress   89–70820
                                                                    CIP

© The American Society for Surgery of the Hand 1990, 1983, 1978

Published and distributed in the United States by Churchill
Livingstone Inc., 1560 Broadway, New York, NY 10036. Distributed
in the United Kingdom by Churchill Livingstone, Robert Stevenson
House, 1–3 Baxter's Place, Leith Walk, Edinburgh EH1 3AF, and by
associated companies, branches, and representatives throughout
the world.

Accurate indications, adverse reactions, and dosage schedules for
drugs are provided in this book, but it is possible that they may
change. The reader is urged to review the package information data
of the manufacturers of the medications mentioned.

Acquisitions Editor: *Leslie Burgess*
Copy Editor: *Kamely Dahir*

Printed in the United States of America

First published in 1990

FOREWORD

The American Society for Surgery of the Hand has always been deeply committed to continuing education. In 1974, a Society task force under the direction of Dr. George E. Omer recognized the need for a concise, compact manual of hand examination and diagnosis, in a format that could be carried in the pocket of a medical student or house officer. The idea was nurtured by Dr. Gordon B. McFarland, the structure developed by Dr. James L. Becton, and the first manuscript written by Dr. Richard I. Burton and edited by Dr. Fred B. Kessler, with input from many other members of the Society.

Over 67,000 copies of that manual have been sold, and the book has also been printed in Japanese and Polish, with plans for translations into several other languages. This third edition has been prepared by Dr. Richard S. Idler and other members of the Hand Surgery Manuals Committee of the American Society for Surgery of the Hand.

The reader will find heavy emphasis on anatomy in this third edition. A thorough knowledge of anatomy is by far the single most important prerequisite for accurate examination and diagnosis of hand and upper extremity problems. It is axiomatic that the best hand surgeons are all good anatomists.

The field of hand surgery is a truly multidisciplinary speciality, for it encompasses the fundamental principles of orthopaedics, plastic surgery, neurosurgery, vascular surgery, microsurgery, and rehabilitation. However, the surgical and technical aspects of hand surgery are only one aspect of this speciality. Meticulous examination and accurate diagnosis still constitute the most important role of any physician dealing with injuries and disorders of the hand.

AMERICAN SOCIETY FOR SURGERY OF THE HAND
David P. Green, M.D.
President, 1988–1989

PREFACE TO THE THIRD EDITION

It has been difficult to improve upon the easily read and comprehended second edition created by Dr. Burton's committee in 1983. It has been one of the best texts on examination and diagnosis of the hand, particularly because it is suitable for use by both new students and old scholars.

Since that is the case, we have retained all of the features of that edition and added several new sections and illustrations. Examinations of the fingertip and nailbed, carpus, and flexor tendon sheath, all newly illustrated, are added to the examination part of the book. There is also new information on the two-point discrimination test and on examination of the circulation.

The diagnosis part of the book now includes sections on fifth CMC fracture-dislocation, scaphoid fractures, the compression test, cubital tunnel syndrome, lateral epicondylitis, congenital constriction band syndrome, and Madelung's deformity.

These revisions and additions reflect our increased understanding of hand anatomy and function, as well as the need to keep pace with the growing sophistication of those who will read and use this information. An attempt has been made to maintain the clarity and efficiency of the original presentation.

The Hand Surgery Manuals Committee would like to thank and compliment those who originally created this text. These individuals made our task an easy one. As Chairman, I would like to thank the members of my committee for their help in this revision. I also greatly appreciate Dr. Lee Dellon's contribution to the revision of the section on sensory nerve anatomy and sensibility testing.

We hope this monograph remains an important reference source for those interested in studying the hand.

Richard S. Idler, M.D.
Chairman, Hand Surgery Manuals Committee, 1989

PREFACE TO THE FIRST EDITION

The hand is composed of material for touch of great sensitivity and a system of exact machinery of great specialization and refinement—all in a most complex array and condensed into a unit weighing less than a pound. With this amazing tool, we implement the desires of the human brain, whether requiring the speed and precision of the fingering hand of a concert violinist or the brute power grasp needed to wield a sledge hammer.

Sir Charles Bell, the leading British anatomist, physiologist, and neurologist of the early 19th century, was among the first to recognize the unique qualities of the human hand: ". . . It is in the human hand that we perceive the consummation of all perfection, as an instrument. This superiority consists in its combination of strength, with variety, extent, and rapidity of motion . . . and the sensibility, which adapt it for holding, pulling, spinning, weaving, and constructing; . . . 'With the hands the laborer supports a family, the parent loves and cares for a baby, the musician plays a sonata, the blind 'read,' and the deaf 'talk.'"[1]

This essential organ, the hand, is often crippled by injury, disease, or birth defects.

To address this human need, there has emerged in the last three decades a special area of expertise—*surgery of the hand*.

One of the earliest pioneers in surgery of the hand was Allen B. Kanavel of Chicago (1874–1938). His main contributions were in the understanding and treatment of infections of the hand, and his book on this subject is a classic. His efforts were furthered by his associate, Sumner Koch (1888–1976).

During this same era, Arthur Steindler (1879–1959) of Iowa City developed the principles and many of the details of tendon and muscle transfers for the disabled upper extremity—concepts which are still used today.

Perhaps the most influential person in the history of surgery of the hand was Sterling Bunnell. In order to improve the treatment of the hands disabled in combat during World War II, he was appointed as a special consultant to the Secretary of War "to guide, integrate, and develop the special field of hand surgery." From the hand centers which he developed sprang a core of surgeons dedicated to the principles and philosophies of Dr. Bunnell.

From this small group of Dr. Bunnell's disciples emerged a group of surgeons from general, orthopaedic, and plastic surgery who, recognizing the uniqueness of this specialized organ, organized the American Society for Surgery of the Hand. Through its influence, in turn, similar hand societies have been founded in most countries of Europe, Asia, and Central and South America. These efforts have culminated in the formation of the International Federation of Societies for Surgery of the Hand.

Today the horizons for surgery of the hand have further expanded to include arthritis, congenital deformities, and even the replantation of amputated parts. As Sterling Bunnell aptly summarized, "to recondition these members successfully is difficult. Surgical reconstruction of the hand requires special careful technique. . . . It is a composite problem requiring the correlation of various specialties — orthopaedic, plastic, and neurologic surgery — the knowledge of any one of which alone is inadequate for repairing the hand. . . . As the problem is composite, the surgeon must also be . . . The surgeon must face the situation and equip himself to handle any and all of the tissues of a limb."[2]

The intent of this brief monograph is to introduce some of the basic anatomic principles upon which is based this new but exacting and essential discipline.

Richard I. Burton, M.D.
Chairman, Instructional Aids Committee, 1979

REFERENCES

1. Bell Sir Charles: The Hand, Its Mechanism and Vital Endowments, as Evincing Design. Coney, Lea and Blanchard, Philadelphia, 1833.
2. Bunnell S: Surgery of the Hand. JB Lippincott, Philadelphia, 1944.

ACKNOWLEDGMENTS

The germinal concept of this book began at a meeting of the Task Force on Continuing Education in 1974 attended by Drs. George Omer, Fred Kessler, James Becton, Edward Nalebuff, and myself. It fell to Dr. Becton to produce a working outline and preliminary drawings of this production. Each chapter was then amplified and supervised by an individual member of the Instructional Aids Committee of the American Society for Surgery of the Hand. Dr. Richard Burton, chairman of that committee, has been tireless in his efforts to produce an academically sound yet practical approach to the physical diagnosis of the hand.

Though this has truly been a product of the entire committee, I am especially grateful to Dr. Becton not only for his original outline, but for his continued efforts; Dr. Burton for his skill and diplomacy in guiding a true committee effort; Dr. Omer for his guidance and Dr. Kessler, without whose spark, continued leadership, and editorial supervision this work might not have been produced at all.

AMERICAN SOCIETY FOR SURGERY OF THE HAND
Gordon B. McFarland, Jr., M.D.
Coordinator, Division of Post-Graduate Education, 1978

CONTENTS

INTRODUCTION

This text is a core of information on the diagnostic history and physical examination of the normal, diseased, or injured hand. A method for thorough, systematic evaluation of the hand is presented so that with practice the reader can develop a routine for accurate examination to achieve a specific diagnosis.

A brief introduction to specific conditions of the hand is given, followed by illustrations of the more common disorders. A limited description of certain lacerations, fractures, dislocations, and deformities is included.

Specific treatment of each diagnosis is *not* discussed. The reader is referred to the standard texts and the current literature of hand surgery for detailed descriptions of treatment methods.

PART 1

EXAMINATION

1

HISTORY AND GENERAL EXAMINATION

HISTORY

Before examining the hands, a detailed history of the present problem should be obtained:

A. What are the patient's age, occupation, and pursuits? Which is the dominant hand? Has there been a previous hand impairment or injury?
B. *In trauma problems,* the history should include the following specific information:

1. *When* did the injury occur and how much time has elapsed since the injury?
2. *Where* did the injury occur? Was it at work, home, or play? Under what conditions was the environment—clean or dirty?
3. *How* did the injury happen? What was the exact mechanism of the injury? (This helps to evaluate the amount of crush, contamination, blood loss, and level of injury to gliding parts.) What was the exact posture of the hand at the time of injury?

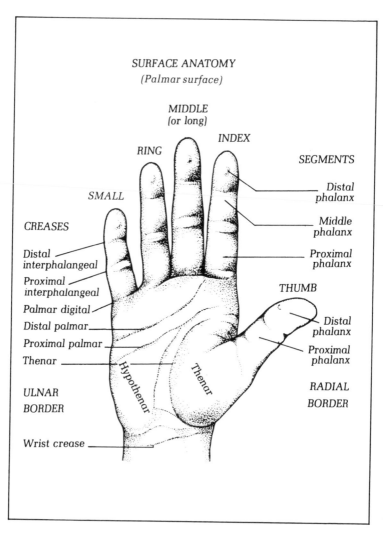

Figure 1
Surface anatomy of the hand

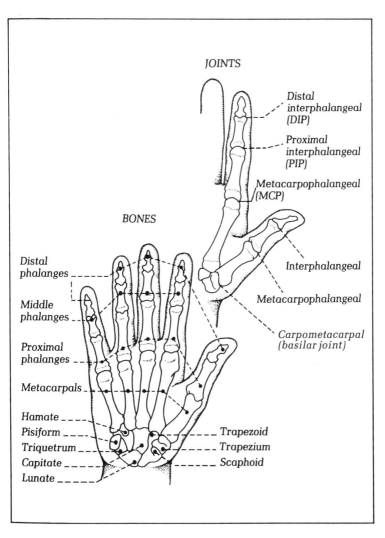

Figure 2
Skeleton of the hand and wrist

   4. *What* previous treatment has been administered?
C. *In nontrauma problems,* particular emphasis should be placed on:
   1. *When* did the pain, sensory change, swelling, or contracture begin? In what sequence? Are these symptoms progressive?
   2. *How* is function impaired in occupation, hobby, and activities of daily living?
   3. *Are* other joints or tendons in this or other extremities painful in a similar way?
   4. *What* activities make the pain worse?
   5. *At what* time of day or night is the pain worse?
D. A review of the past medical history and a review of systems should be obtained as part of the complete evaluation of the hand.

TERMINOLOGY

In order to avoid confusion it is important that standard terminology for structures of the hand be used. The hand and digits have a dorsal surface, a volar or palmar surface, and radial and ulnar borders (Fig. 1). The palm is divided into the thenar, mid-palm, and hypothenar areas. The names of the digits are the thumb, index, middle (long), ring, and small fingers. The thenar mass or eminence is that muscular area on the palmar surface overlying the thumb metacarpal. The hypothenar is that muscle mass on the palmar surface overlying the small finger metacarpal. Each finger has three joints: the metacarpophalangeal (MCP), the proximal interphalangeal (PIP), and the distal interphalangeal (DIP) joints (Fig. 2). Note the location of the finger MCP joints in the palm near the distal palmar crease, with the palmar-digital creases and finger webs at the level of the middle third of the proximal phalanges.

The thumb has an MCP and only one interphalangeal (IP) joint. The carpometacarpal (CMC) joint of the thumb is particularly important because of its mobility. There are proximal, middle, and distal phalanges in the fingers and only a proximal and a distal phalanx in the thumb.

The terminology used to describe the motion of the joints is illustrated in Figure 3.

PHYSICAL EXAMINATION (see Ch. 2 for details)

The entire upper extremity should be exposed and evaluated when the hand is examined. Assessment of active shoulder motion, elbow motion, and pronation and supination of the forearm is essential. Motion of these joints is necessary for proper positioning of the hand for function. Any discrepancy between active and passive mobility should be noted.

When inspecting the hand, one should observe its color to assess circulation as well as the radial and ulnar pulses. The presence of swelling or edema should be noted as well as any abnormal posture or position. Skin moisture, localized tenderness, and sensibility must be evaluated.

After injury to the hand there is often secondary stiffness and limited range of motion (ROM) of other joints of the extremity as well as the part involved. The range of both passive and active motion of the wrist, MCP joint, and IP joints of each digit should be measured and recorded. Grip and pinch strength should also be documented. The patient's ability to use the hand for simple function should be evaluated.

Accurate recording of the findings of the examination of the hand is most important. A simple sketch of the hand with appropriate notations and measurements is often very helpful.

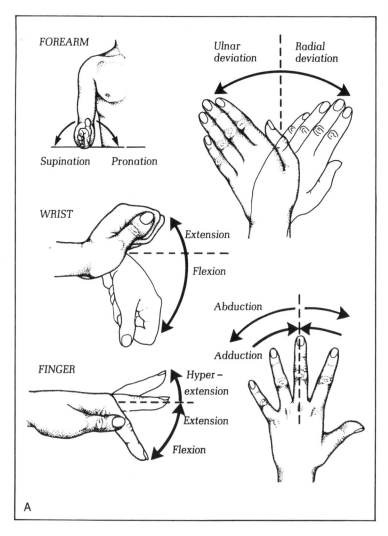

Figure 3
Terminology of hand and digit motion

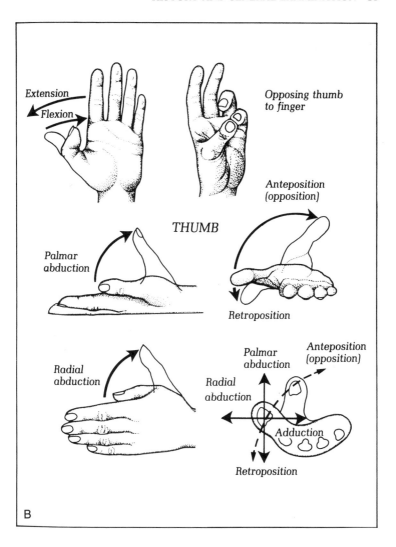

B

Subsequent re-examination of the hand is just as important as the initial examination and should be done each time the patient returns for follow-up. Only by making appropriate serial recordings during the follow-up period can the examiner know for certain whether or not there is improvement in the patient's condition.

2

EXAMINATION OF SPECIFIC SYSTEMS

SKIN

The normal palmar skin is thick, tethered, irregularly surfaced, and moist, providing for traction and durability. Normal skin on the dorsum of the hand is thin and mobile, permitting motion of the various joints. The dorsum of the hand is the common site of edema, which may limit flexion. The examiner should note the presence or absence of swelling, wrinkles, color, moisture, scars, skin lesions, and surface irregularities.

THE FINGERTIP AND NAILBED

The fingertip is defined as that portion of the digit distal to the insertion of the extensor and flexor tendons into the base of the distal phalanx (Fig. 4). The tuft of the distal phalanx is well-padded by adipose tissue and covered by highly innervated skin which is tethered to the distal phalanx through a series of fibrosepta. The nailbed complex on the dorsum of the fingertip is important in providing additional stabilization of the palmar soft tissues against compression and shear forces (Fig. 4). The nailbed complex is also called the perionychium. The

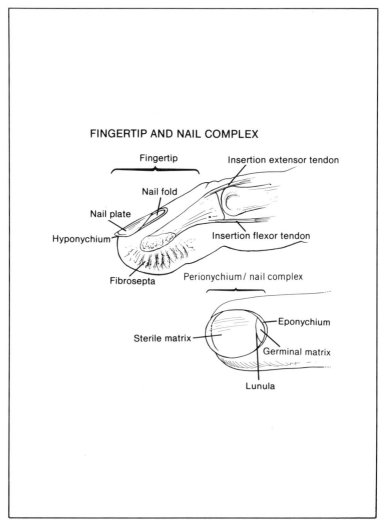

Figure 4
The fingertip and nail complex

distal skin of the nailbed complex is referred to as the hyponychium. The cuticle or thin layer of skin bridging the nail plate to the dorsal skin of the nail complex is referred to as the eponychium. The nail plate arises from a pocket called the nail fold. The floor of the nail plate or nailbed is comprised of the proximal germinal matrix and distal sterile matrix. The semicircular division between these two areas is called the lunula.

MUSCLES

The muscles that power the hand may be divided into extrinsic and intrinsic muscles. The *extrinsic muscles* have their muscle bellies in the forearm and their tendon insertions in the hand. They are further divided into extrinsic flexor and extensor muscles. The flexors are on the volar surface of the forearm and flex the wrist and digits; the extensors are on the dorsum of the forearm and extend the wrist and digits.

The *intrinsic muscles* have their origins and insertions within the hand.

These muscles should be systematically evaluated. Ask the patient to "make a fist" and "straighten out your fingers"; this gives the examiner a general idea of the active ROM of the digits. However, it is necessary to examine each muscle group specifically.

Specific extrinsic muscle testing

Extrinsic flexor muscles

The function of the *flexor pollicis longus (FPL)* muscle, whose tendon inserts on the volar base of the distal

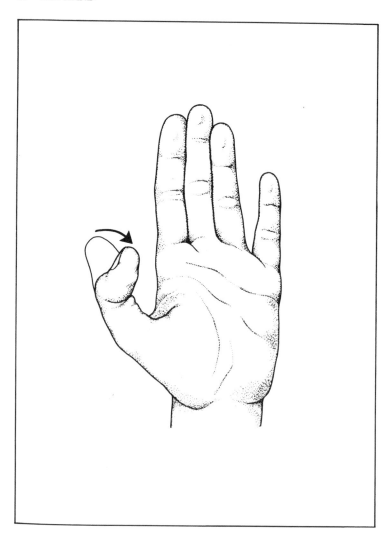

Figure 5
Testing for FPL musculotendinous function

phalanx of the thumb, can be evaluated by asking the patient to "bend the tip of your thumb" (Fig. 5). The muscle strength is tested against resistance supplied by the examiner.

The *flexor digitorum profundus (FDP)* can be tested by asking the patient to "bend the tip of your finger" (Fig. 6). The PIP joint is stabilized in extension by the examiner as the distal joint is actively flexed. As each finger is examined, the muscle is tested against resistance.

Each *flexor digitorum superficialis (FDS)* is individually tested by asking the patient to "bend your finger at the middle joint" (Fig. 7). The other fingers must be stabilized in extension by the examiner so as to block profundus function. (The profundus tendons of the ulnar three digits share a common muscle belly, and thus independent flexion of any finger with the other digits restrained in extension requires intact FDS musculotendinous functions to that finger.) The procedure is repeated for each finger.

The *flexor carpi ulnaris (FCU)*, *flexor carpi radialis (FCR)*, and *palmaris longus (PL)* are evaluated by asking the patient to flex his wrist while the examiner palpates the tendons of these muscles. The FCU inserts into the pisiform and the FCR into the volar aspect of the index metacarpal. The PL inserts into the palmar fascia. The PL will be noted to lie between the FCR radially and FCU ulnarly on the volar surface of the wrist during this maneuver, especially if the thumb is simultaneously opposed to the small finger.

Extrinsic extensor muscles

The extrinsic extensor muscle bellies of the hand overlie the dorsum of the forearm, and their tendons pass over the

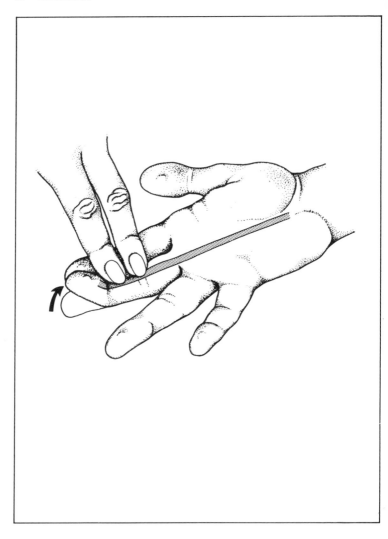

Figure 6
Testing for FDP musculotendinous function

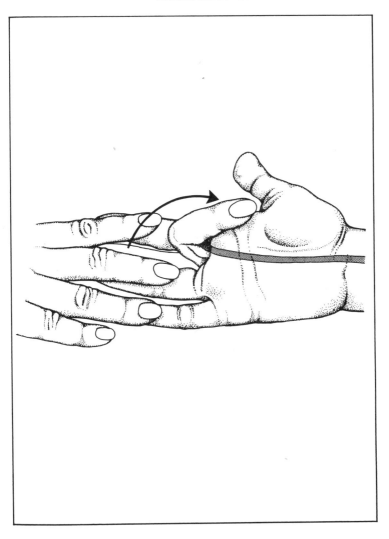

Figure 7
Testing FDS musculotendinous function

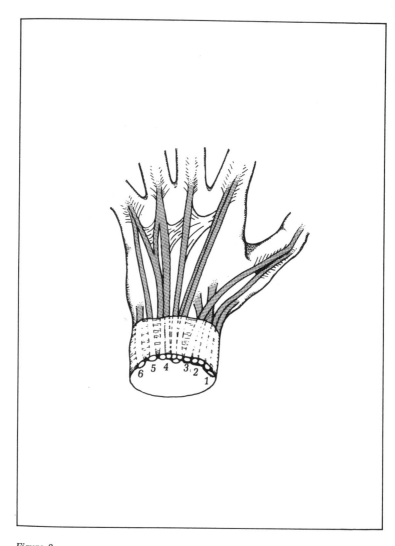

Figure 8
Arrangement of extensor tendons at the wrist into six compartments:
dorsal and cross-sectional views

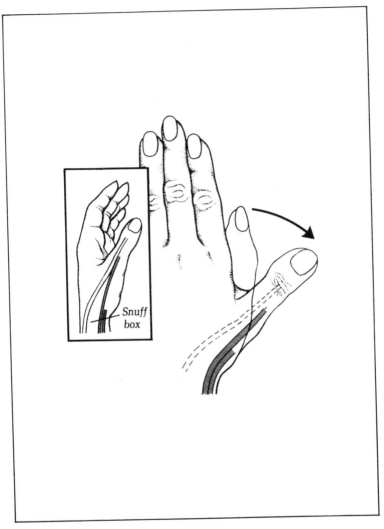

Snuff
box

Figure 9
Testing for EPB and APL musculotendinous function

dorsum of the wrist to insert in the hand (Fig. 8). They are arranged in six tendon compartments over the dorsum of the wrist. A systematic examination of the tendons passing through each compartment is done.

The *first dorsal wrist compartment* contains the tendons of the *abductor pollicis longus (APL)*, which inserts at the dorsal base of the thumb metacarpal, and the *extensor pollicis brevis (EPB)*, which inserts at the dorsal base of the proximal phalanx of the thumb. These are evaluated by asking the patient to "bring your thumb out to the side" (Fig. 9). The examiner can palpate the taut tendons over the radial side of the wrist going to the thumb.

The *second dorsal wrist compartment* contains the tendons of the *extensor carpi radialis longus (ECRL)* and the *extensor carpi radialis brevis (ECRB)* muscles (Fig.10). They insert at the dorsal base of the index and middle metacarpals, respectively. These are evaluated by asking the patient to "make a fist and bring your wrist back strongly." The examiner can give resistance and palpate the tendons over the dorsoradial aspect of the wrist.

In the *third dorsal wrist compartment*, the *extensor pollicis longus (EPL)* tendon passes around Lister's tubercle of the radius and inserts on the dorsal base of the distal phalanx of the thumb. This muscle is evaluated by placing the hand flat on the table and having the patient lift only the thumb off the surface (Fig. 11).

The *fourth dorsal wrist compartment* contains the tendons that are the MCP joint extensors of the fingers (Figs. 8 and 12). The *extensor digitorum communis (EDC)* and the *extensor indicis proprius (EIP)* muscle tendons are evaluated by asking the patient to "straighten your fingers" and by observing MCP joint extension.

The EIP tendon can be isolated on examination by asking the patient to "bring your pointing finger out

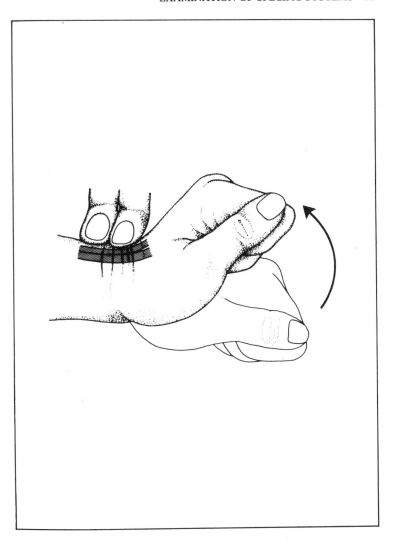

Figure 10
Testing for ECRL and ECRB musculotendinous function

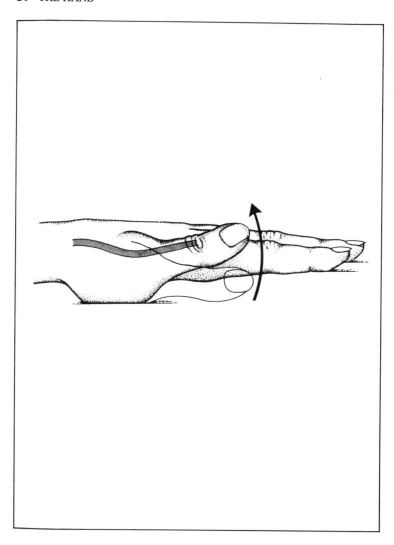

Figure 11
Testing for EPL musculotendinous function

straight, with the other fingers bent in a fist." The EIP is acting alone to extend the index finger MCP joint (Fig. 12).

The *fifth dorsal wrist compartment* contains the tendon of the *extensor digiti minimi (EDM)* (Fig. 12). This is evaluated by asking the patient to "straighten out your small finger with your other fingers bent in a fist." This extends the MCP joint of the small finger. The EDM is acting alone to extend the small finger.

The *sixth dorsal wrist compartment* contains the tendon of the *extensor carpi ulnaris (ECU)*, which inserts at the dorsal base of the fifth metacarpal (Fig. 13). This is evaluated by asking the patient to "pull your hand up and out to the side." The taut tendon can be palpated over the ulnar side of the wrist just distal to the ulnar head.

Extrinsic extensor tightness. The extensor tendons can become adherent over the dorsum of the hand or wrist, limiting finger flexion. This can be tested by maintaining the wrist in neutral and passively extending the MCP joint and flexing the PIP joint. Normally, the PIP joint should flex. The test is then repeated with the MCP joint passively flexed. If the PIP joint will passively flex when the MCP joint is extended, but will not flex readily with the MCP joint flexed, the adherent extrinsic extensors are checkreining the simultaneous flexion of finger MCP and PIP joints. This is called "extrinsic extensor tightness."

Intrinsic muscles

The intrinsic muscles of the hand are those that have their origins and insertions within the hand. These are the thenar muscle group, *adductor pollicis (AdP)*, lumbrical, and interosseous muscles and the hypothenar muscle group.

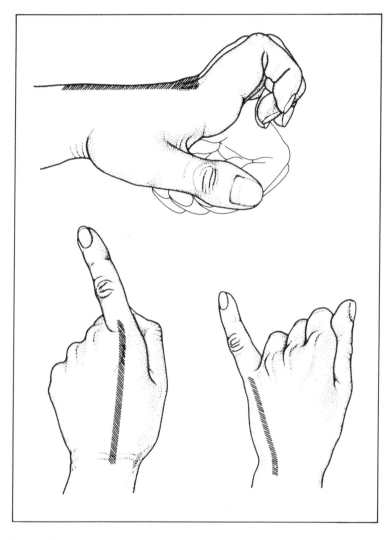

Figure 12
Testing for EDC, EIP, and EDM musculotendinous function

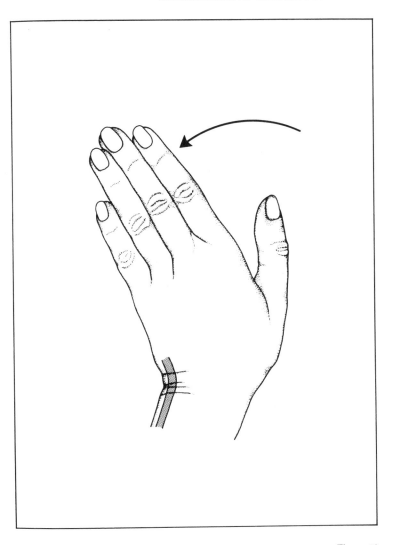

Figure 13
Testing for ECU musculotendinous function

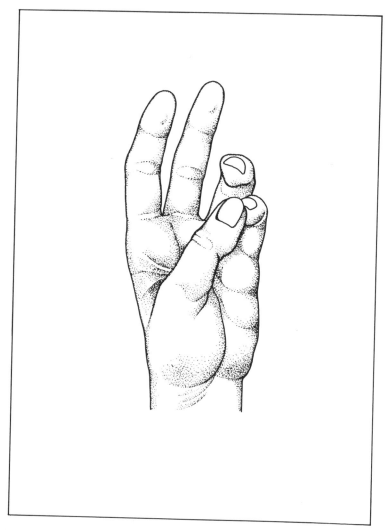

Figure 14
Testing for thumb opposition

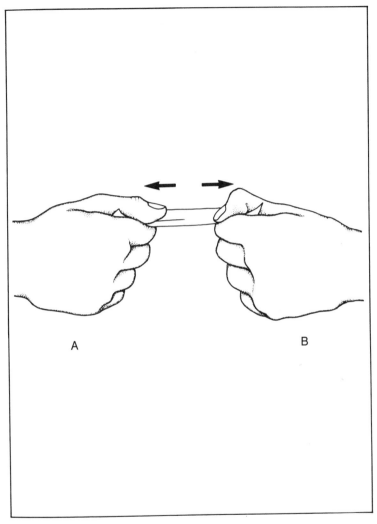

A

B

Figure 15 (A&B)
Froment's sign is positive in hand B

The thenar muscles

The thenar muscles are the muscles covering the thumb metacarpal. They are the *abductor pollicis brevis (APB)*, *opponens pollicis (OP)*, and *flexor pollicis brevis (FPB)*. These muscles pronate or oppose the thumb (see Fig. 3) and can be evaluated by asking the patient to "touch the thumb and small fingertips together so that the nails are parallel" (Fig. 14). They can also be tested by asking the patient to place the dorsum of the hand flat on the table and raise the thumb up straight to form a 90° angle with the palm (see Fig. 3). At that time it is most important to palpate the thenar muscles to note if they contract. It is helpful to examine and compare the contralateral hand in a similar way to detect slight variations in muscle mass and function. The thenar muscles are usually innervated by the motor branch of the median nerve. In some patients, however, the thenar muscles may be partially innervated by the ulnar nerve.

The adductor pollicis muscle

Thumb adduction is separately tested by having the patient forcibly hold a piece of paper between the thumb and radial side of the index proximal phalanx (Fig. 15). The muscle that powers this motion is the AdP, which is innervated by the ulnar nerve. When this muscle is weak or nonfunctioning, the thumb IP joint flexes with this maneuver (Froment's sign). In this evaluation the two hands must be compared.

The interosseous and lumbrical muscles

The interosseous and lumbrical muscles act on the fingers to flex the MCP joints and extend the IP joints. The interosseous muscles also abduct and adduct the fingers. The interosseous muscles, which lie on either side of the finger metacarpals, are innervated by the ulnar nerve. They can be evaluated by asking the patient to "spread your fingers apart" while the examiner palpates the first dorsal interosseous to see if it contracts. In another test, with the hand flat on a table, the patient is asked to elevate (i.e., hyperextend the MCP joint with the IP joints straight) the middle finger and radially and ulnarly deviate it (Fig. 16). (This eliminates the extrinsic extensors, which some patients can use to mimic interossei finger abduction-adduction.)

The hypothenar muscles

The hypothenar muscles —*abductor digiti minimi (ADM)*, *flexor digiti minimi (FDM)*, and *opponens digiti minimi (ODM)* —are evaluated as a group by asking the patient to "bring the small finger away from the other fingers" (Fig. 17). This muscle mass is palpated at that time, and a dimpling of the hypothenar skin is noted.

Intrinsic muscle tightness. To test for finger intrinsic muscle tightness the MCP joint of the finger is held in extension (0° neutral position) while the PIP joint is passively flexed by the examiner (Fig. 18). The MCP joint is then flexed and the PIP joint is passively flexed in the same manner as before. If the PIP joint can be passively flexed with the MCP joint in flexion, but cannot be fully flexed when the MCP joint is extended, there is tightness of the intrinsic muscles. This is called "intrinsic tightness."

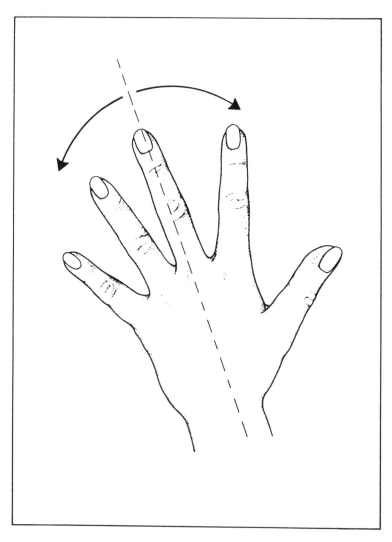

Figure 16
Testing for interosseous muscle function

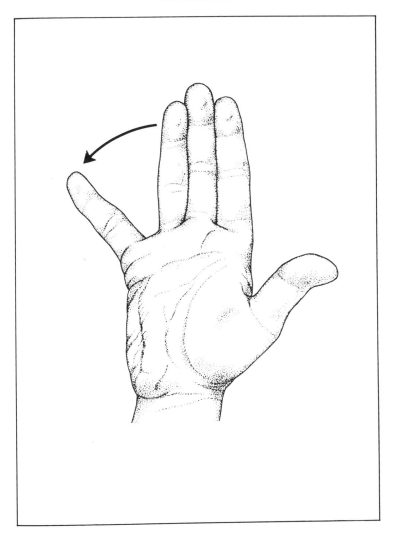

Figure 17
Testing for hypothenar muscle function

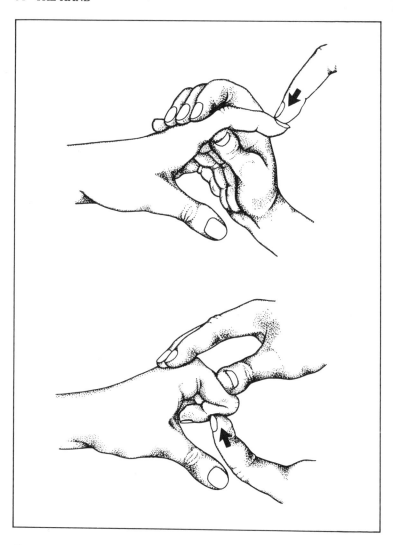

Figure 18
Intrinsic muscle tightness

NERVES

The hand is innervated by the median, ulnar, and radial nerves. Each of the three major nerves passes through a muscle in the forearm and each passes points of potential entrapment. All three nerves are involved in control of the wrist, fingers, and thumb.

The median nerve

The median nerve enters the forearm through the pronator teres muscle and innervates the following muscles: pronator teres, FCR, PL, FDS, radial part of the FDP, FPL, and pronator quadratus (Fig. 19). The branch of the median nerve that innervates the latter three muscles is referred to as the anterior interosseous nerve. The median nerve travels distally through the forearm between the FDS and FDP muscles. It enters the hand through the carpal tunnel accompanied by the nine extrinsic flexor tendons of the digits. The thenar motor branch innervates the APB, the superficial belly of the FPB (variably so), and the OP. The common digital branches innervate the lumbrical muscles to the index and long fingers. The nerve then continues through the palm as sensory branches (described below).

The ulnar nerve

The ulnar nerve enters the forearm from the posterior to the medial epicondyle of the humerus and passes between

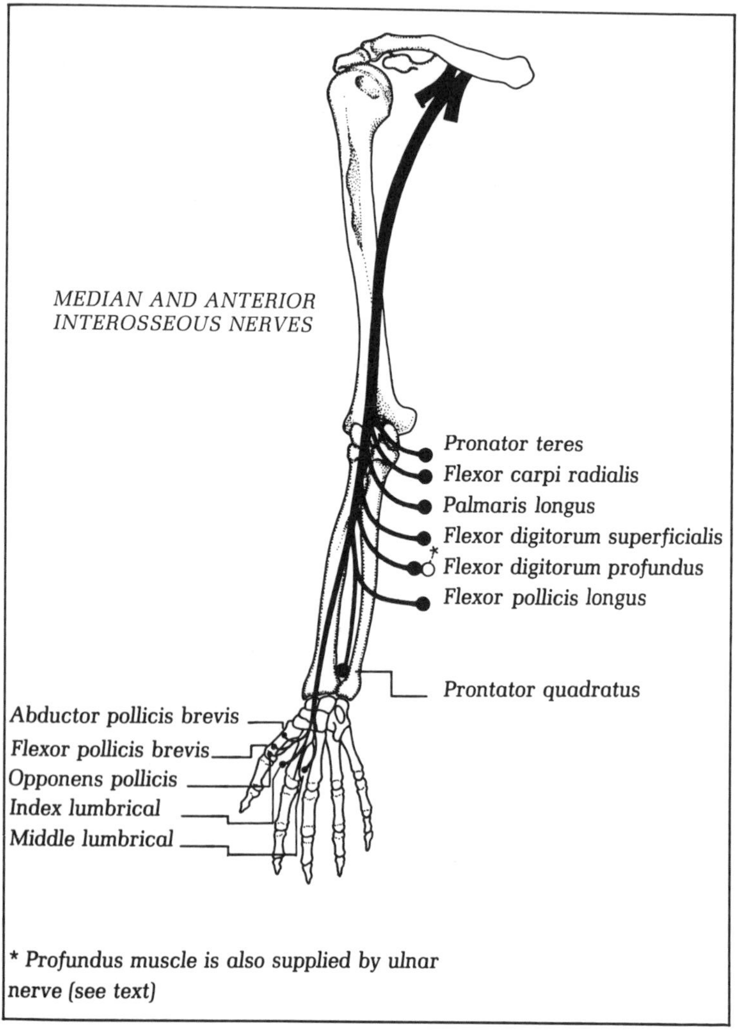

Figure 19
Muscles innervated by the median and anterior interosseous nerves in the forearm and hand

the two heads of the FCU (Fig. 20). It innervates the following muscles in the forearm: the FCU and the ulnar part of the FDP (usually to the ring and small fingers, occasionally to the long finger). It enters the hand at the wrist accompanied by the ulnar artery through a tunnel radial to the pisiform bone, ulnar to the hook of the hamate, volar to the deep transverse carpal ligament, and dorsal to the volar carpal ligament (Fig. 21). This tunnel is known as the ulnar tunnel or Guyon's canal. The ulnar nerve innervates the hypothenar muscles (the ADM, FDM, ODM), the seven interosseous muscles, the lumbrical muscles to the ring and small fingers, and the AdP. It may innervate part or all of the FPB.

The radial nerve

The radial nerve innervates the triceps, anconeus, brachioradialis, and ECRL muscles above the elbow and ECRB as the nerve enters the forearm (Fig. 22). It passes through the supinator muscle to innervate the following muscles in the forearm: supinator, EDC, EDM, ECU, APL, EPL, EPB, and EIP. Thus its important motor function is to innervate the muscles in the forearm that extend the wrist and MCP joints and that abduct and extend the thumb. No intrinsic muscles in the hand are innervated by the radial nerve.

Sensory branches of the nerves

As it leaves the carpal tunnel, the *median nerve* divides into common sensory branches, which subsequently divide and innervate the palmar surface of the thumb, the index and middle fingers, and the radial side of the ring

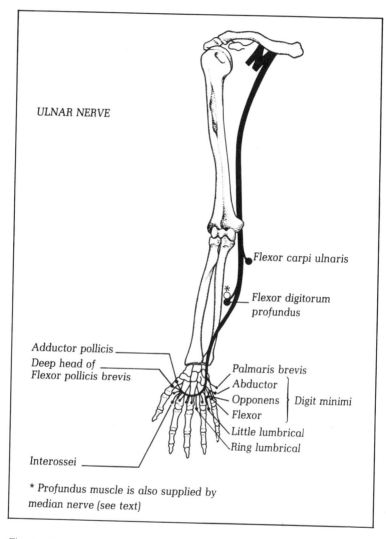

ULNAR NERVE

Flexor carpi ulnaris

*
Flexor digitorum
profundus

Adductor pollicis
Deep head of
Flexor pollicis brevis

Palmaris brevis
Abductor
Opponens } Digit minimi
Flexor
Little lumbrical
Ring lumbrical

Interossei

* Profundus muscle is also supplied by
median nerve (see text)

Figure 20
Muscles innervated by the ulnar nerve in the forearm and hand

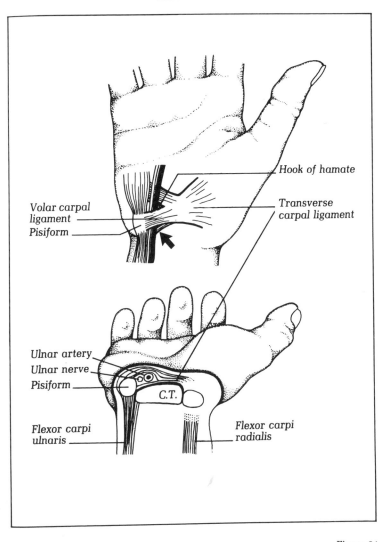

Figure 21

Ulnar tunnel at wrist (Guyon's canal) contains ulnar artery and nerve; CT, carpal tunnel

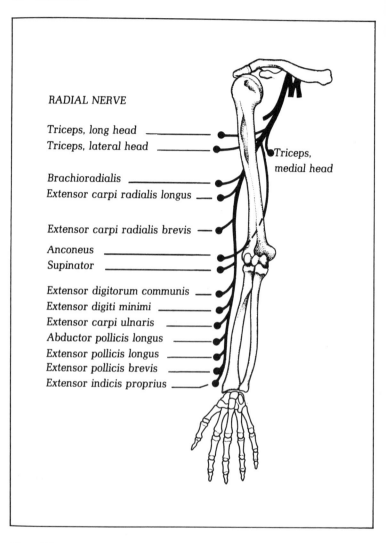

RADIAL NERVE

Triceps, long head _____

Triceps, lateral head _____

Triceps, medial head

Brachioradialis _____

Extensor carpi radialis longus __

Extensor carpi radialis brevis —

Anconeus _____

Supinator _____

Extensor digitorum communis __

Extensor digiti minimi _____

Extensor carpi ulnaris _____

Abductor pollicis longus _____

Extensor pollicis longus _____

Extensor pollicis brevis _____

Extensor indicis proprius _____

Figure 22
Muscles innervated by the radial nerve in the forearm and hand

finger (Fig. 23). Dorsal digital branches arise from the digital branches to innervate distal to the PIP joint, the dorsal aspect of the index and middle fingers, and the radial half of the ring finger. The median nerve also innervates the volar wrist capsule by the terminal branch of the anterior interosseous nerve.

The *ulnar nerve* divides distal to the hook of the hamate into digital branches and innervates the small finger and the ulnar half of the ring finger (Fig. 23). The dorsal cutaneous branch of the ulnar nerve enters the dorsal aspect of the hand over the small and ring metacarpals, the dorsum of the small finger, and dorso-ulnar half of the ring finger.

The *radial nerve* supplies sensibility to the radial three quarters of the dorsum of the hand and the dorsum of the thumb (Fig. 23). It also supplies sensibility to the dorsum of the index and middle fingers and the radial half of the ring finger as far distally as the PIP joint of each. It also innervates the dorsal wrist capsule by the terminal branch of the posterior interosseous nerve.

Anatomic variation

Anatomic variation should be considered in all cases where there has been an injury to a major nerve trunk. For example, there can be variations in the distribution of the ulnar and median nerves in the hand. The entire ring finger and ulnar side of the long finger may be innervated by the ulnar nerve, or the entire ring finger may be innervated by the median nerve. The palmar aspect of the thumb may be innervated by the radial nerve. The lateral antebrachial cutaneous nerve frequently overlaps the radial sensory nerve.

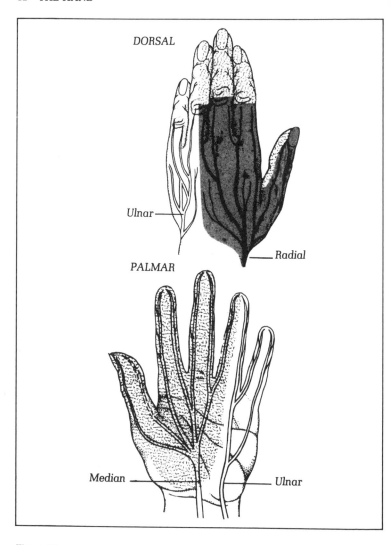

Figure 23
Distribution of major nerves innervating the hand for sensory function

Sensibility

Sensibility is one of the most important functions of the hand. The insensible hand is poorly used even when the tendons and joints are normal.

Normal skin should be slightly moist. Nerve dysfunction causes loss of sympathetic innervation in the area of distribution, and the skin becomes dry. This is of clinical help in evaluating nerve dysfunction. Testing the finger with a sharp-pointed object, such as a pin, or thermal testing is not as critical and helpful as to test it for tactile gnosis by the moving and static two-point light touch discrimination test (2PD). In this test the hand is positioned at rest on a flat firm surface and the patient closes his eyes. A device that measures innervation density, such as the Disk-Criminator or something as simple as a bent paper clip (Fig. 24) is used by beginning at a 6-mm distance between the prongs and proceeding higher or lower to determine the critical distance at which the patient indicates he can distinguish two points from one. An abnormal value (>6 mm static or >3 mm moving 2PD) indicates axonal loss and is the sensory system equivalent of wasting or atrophy in the motor system. This will occur with all nerve division and severe nerve compression. Vibratory perception is also lost with nerve division. With a mild or moderate degree of nerve compression, 2PD is preserved but sensory threshold changes, such as diminished perception of tuning fork stimulation and abnormal cutaneous pressure threshold (Semmes-Weinstein monofilament testing), occur.

In evaluating children for traumatic nerve injuries, it may not be possible or practical to perform a 2PD test. In this situation, the use of the "immersion test" may be of benefit. The innervated glabrous skin of the hand will wrinkle on immersion in water for 5 to 10 minutes.

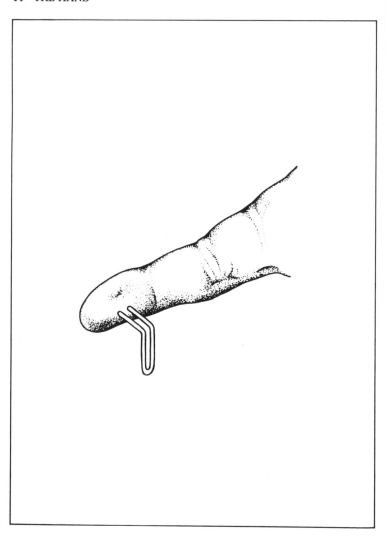

Figure 24
Two-point discrimination testing

Failure of the skin to wrinkle should raise the suspicion of an underlying nerve injury.

CIRCULATION

The radial and ulnar arteries supply the hand with blood. There is an arterial arch system that gives the hand a generous collateral blood supply (Fig. 25).

The circulation of the hand is evaluated by noting the color of the skin and fingernails as well as the blanching and flush of the nailbed. The Allen test, used to determine patency of the arteries supplying the hand, is done as follows (Fig. 25):

1. Compress the radial and ulnar arteries at the wrist.
2. Have the patient make a fist, open and close it several times to exsanguinate the hand, and then open the hand again into a relaxed position (avoid hyperextension at this point, as it will maintain blanching).
3. Release the radial artery only. If the palm and all five digits fill with blood, then the radial artery is patent, with good collateral flow into the ulnar artery system.
4. Repeat steps 1 and 2.
5. Release the ulnar artery only. If the entire hand flushes, then the ulnar artery is patent, with good flow into the radial system.
6. Normal filling-time for the hand through either artery is usually under 5 seconds. A distinct difference in filling-time may suggest the dominance of one artery in providing circulation to the hand.

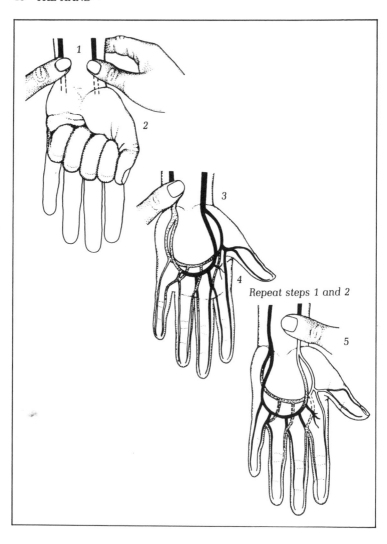

Figure 25
Allen test for arterial patency

The Allen test can also be carried out on a single digit by expressing the blood out of the digit and occluding both digital arteries and then releasing the radial digital artery and noting the filling of the digit. The same procedure is carried out on the ulnar digital artery. This will help to evaluate the patency of each digital vessel to that finger.

Another means of evaluating the arterial circulation of the hand is the Doppler probe. This device is readily available in most emergency rooms. The device can be used to confirm the presence of pulsatile flow and to map out the course of arteries through the hand.

ANATOMY OF THE BONES AND JOINTS

The skeleton of the hand consists of 27 bones, divided into three groups: the carpus, the metacarpal bones, and the phalanges (see Fig. 2).

The carpus

The eight carpal bones are divided into two rows. Those in the proximal row, beginning from the radial side, are the scaphoid, lunate, triquetrum, and pisiform. Those in the distal row are the trapezium, trapezoid, capitate, and hamate. Much of the surface of the carpal bones is covered with cartilage, with roughened areas dorsally and volarly for ligamentous attachments and for entry of the vascular supply to the bone.

Wrist flexion and extension as well as radial and ulnar deviation result from radiocarpal and intercarpal motion, whereas pronation and supination occur through the proximal and distal radioulnar joints.

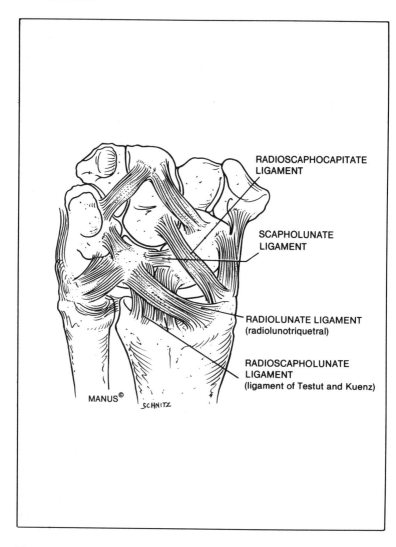

Figure 26
Palmar view of stabilizing ligaments of the radiocarpal joint

The versatile ROM of the wrist and its stability are provided by a well-developed system of ligaments interconnecting the carpus and radius. These are most highly developed on the palmar aspect of the wrist. The important ligaments stabilizing the radial aspect of the carpus are the scapholunate interosseous ligament, radioscaphocapitate ligament, and radioscapholunate ligament (Fig. 26). On the ulnar side of the wrist, the primary stabilizer of the radioulnar joint is the triangular fibrocartilage, which originates from the dorso-ulnar corner of the distal radius and inserts at the base of the ulnar styloid (Fig. 27). The triangular fibrocartilage together with ulnolunate ligament and the ulnar collateral ligament comprise the ulnocarpal complex, which stabilizes the ulnar aspect of the carpus.

A number of clinical tests can be used to evaluate the stability of the wrist. The piano key test evaluates the distal radioulnar joint. With one hand, firmly stabilize the distal radius; with the other hand, grasp the head of the ulna between the thumb and index fingers. Evaluate the freedom of motion in an anteroposterior plane as well as pain and crepitance. The scaphoid shift maneuver is performed by placing the examiner's thumb over the palmar aspect of the distal pole of the scaphoid. A constant pressure is maintained with the examining thumb as the wrist is moved from a position of extension, ulnar deviation to flexion, radial deviation, and back again. The presence of dorsal wrist pain or a clunk suggests possible instability of the scapholunate ligament. The lunotriquetral shear maneuver involves stabilizing the lunate between the thumb and index finger of one hand and the triquetrum between the thumb and index finger of the other hand. A shear stress is then created in an anteroposterior plane between these two bones. Discomfort in this area suggests the possibility of

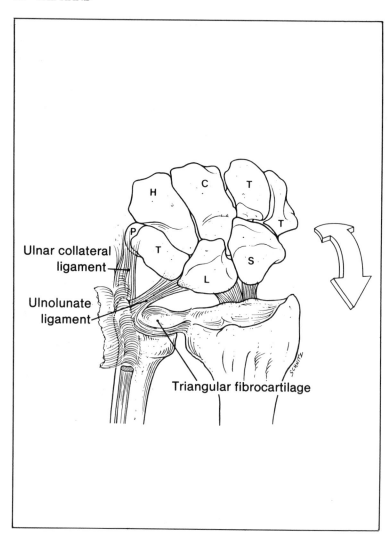

Figure 27
Stabilizing ligaments of the ulnocarpal joint

injury to the lunotriquetral interosseous ligament. In performing all of these manuevers, it is important to repeat the test on the uninjured, opposite wrist to provide a basis for comparison of the patient's symptoms.

It is important to emphasize that the hand is not flat. It is based on a system of skeletal arches which must be maintained to preserve hand function (Fig. 28).

Fixed and mobile units

The metacarpals of the index and long fingers are firmly attached to the rigidly interconnected distal carpal row to form the "fixed" unit of the hand. From this are suspended the "mobile or adaptive" components of the hand — the thumb, the entire ring and small rays (including metacarpals), and the phalanges of the index and long fingers.

The longitudinal arch is apparent in the lateral projection and is formed by the metacarpals and phalanges. There are two transverse arches: the proximal arch at the distal carpus and the distal arch at the metacarpal heads.

The thumb metacarpal articulates with the trapezium, forming the unique basilar joint, which allows for a wide latitude of thumb motion (Figs. 3 and 29).

The MCP and IP joints of the fingers are stabilized on both sides by collateral ligaments and anteriorly by a palmar fibrocartilaginous "volar" plate (Fig. 30).The digital flexor tendons lie just anterior to these plates. The configuration of the metacarpal heads causes their collateral ligaments to be slack in extension, permitting abduction, adduction, and circumduction. In flexion, however, MCP collateral ligaments become taut, providing stability to the joint.

Articular configuration of the IP joints and the geometry of the collateral ligaments do not allow significant

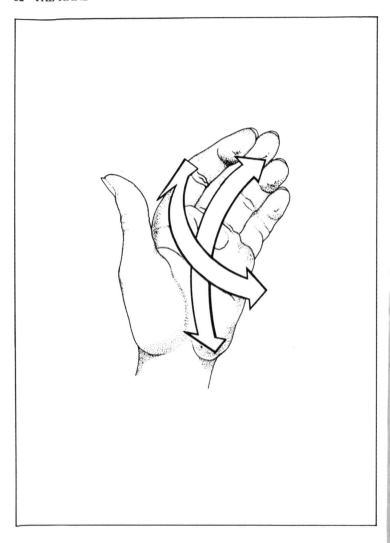

Figure 28
Arches of the hand

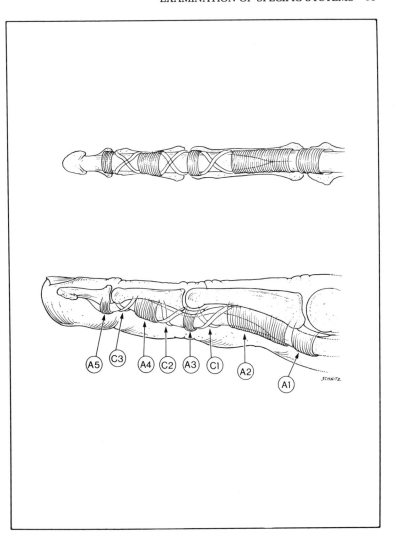

Figure 31
Pulleys of the digital flexor sheath; A, annular pulleys;
C, cruciate pulleys

mediolateral motion in extension or in flexion. The MCP joint of the thumb is more like the hinged IP joints than the freely movable MCP joints of the fingers.

At the level of the MCP joint, the flexor tendons of the digits enter a fibro-osseous tunnel referred to as the flexor sheath. At specific sites, the sheath is thickened by annular fibers called pulleys (Fig. 31). The function of the flexor sheath is to stabilize the tendons closely against the palmar surface of the phalanges, facilitate efficient excursion of the tendons, and provide for tendon nutrition. In the fingers, the A2 and A4 pulleys are most important for maintaining the integrity of finger flexion. Without these two pulleys, the fingertip cannot be brought to the distal palmar flexion crease with normal tendor excursion. The flexor tendons and inner wall of the sheath are lined with a tissue called tenosynovium. This tissue is important in minimizing the friction of tendon excursion as well as in providing tendon nutrition through the process of diffusion.

PART 2

COMMON CLINICAL PROBLEMS

3

LACERATIONS

One should develop a routine for examining the patient with a lacerated forearm or hand so that nerve and tendon injuries will not be overlooked. The patient who presents with a bleeding laceration of the hand should be asked to lie down. The hand is elevated, a sterile dressing is used to cover the wound, and gentle direct pressure is applied. The bleeding will usually stop within a few minutes. The practice of "clamping a bleeder" in a lacerated hand should be avoided. Previously undamaged vital structures, such as nerve or tendon, may be inadvertently crushed and irrevocably damaged in an unnecessary attempt to clamp a blood vessel.

There is a tendency on the part of inexperienced physicians to look into the wound and see if nerves or tendons have been cut. However, much more can be learned on the initial examination by covering the wound and performing a gentle, systematic examination of the forearm and hand *distal* to the injury (Fig. 32). Each flexor tendon must be tested separately for function, and it is important to test IP function against gentle resistance. A partially cut tendon may be able to flex the finger, but it will not be able to do so against resistance without causing pain.

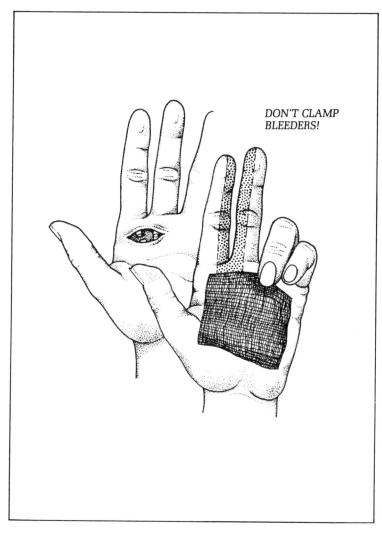

Figure 32
Examination of the lacerated hand

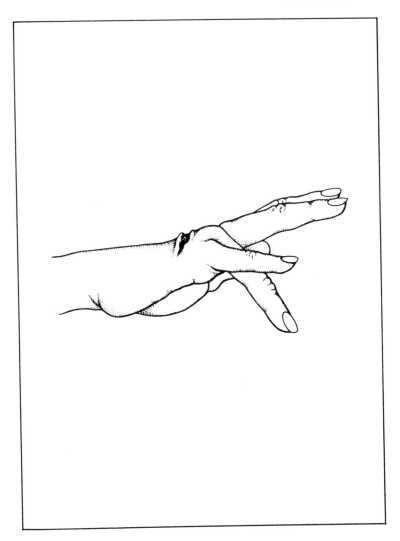

Figure 33
Laceration of EDC over MCP joint (i.e., distal to juncturae tendinae)

The position of the unsupported fingers should be noted. When the flexor tendon is completely severed, the unsupported finger rests in extension (Fig. 32); when the extrinsic extensor tendon is completely severed, the unsupported finger rests in flexion (Fig. 33). A careful distal sensory examination is then done. In the emergency room setting, especially with a frightened child, far more can be learned about the presence or absence of sensation using a light touch with a wisp of cotton than by testing sharp/dull with a pin. Only after the hand has been completely assessed by the examining physician should any anesthetic be used.

In lacerations of the dorsal aspect of the MCP joint of the finger, a severed EDC will preclude active extension of the MCP joint (Fig. 33).

Note that the intact intrinsic muscles will actively extend the IP joints in the absence of extrinsic extensor tendon function, just as the intact intrinsic muscles will actively flex the MCP joint in the absence of extrinsic flexor tendon function.

A laceration over the MCP joint (knuckles) should alert the examiner to the possibility of its having resulted from a human bite or a blow against some teeth. These lacerations are of special importance because of the risk of severe infection.

A radiograph of the hand in the anteroposterior, lateral, and oblique views should be done to check for debris that may be embedded beneath the skin. Some glass is radiopaque and will therefore be shown on the film. However, some glass, wood, and plastic may not be radiopaque and may not be seen on the film.

Associated fractures should be ruled out.

4

COMMON FRACTURES AND DISLOCATIONS

Fractures of the bones of the hand are classified by the nature and site of the fracture line and whether the fracture is closed or open (Fig. 34). An open fracture is one that communicates with the skin wound.

Because of angular or rotational deformity, simple inspection of the hand will often alert the examiner that a bone or joint injury has occurred. It is important that proper anteroposterior and true lateral radiographs be obtained to confirm the presence of bony injury; the amount of angulation of the fracture may not be appreciated on improperly positioned views. A careful physical examination is essential to evaluate rotational alignment. Since the flexed fingers normally point toward the tubercle of the scaphoid, malrotation is best evaluated by observing the fingers in this position. The rotational alignment of the involved finger can also be compared with that of adjacent uninjured fingers by noting if the planes of the distal fingernails are parallel.

It is important to realize that the deformity of fractures in the hand is due not only to the mechanism of injury but also to the deforming forces of the musculotendinous units acting across the fracture site (Fig. 35).

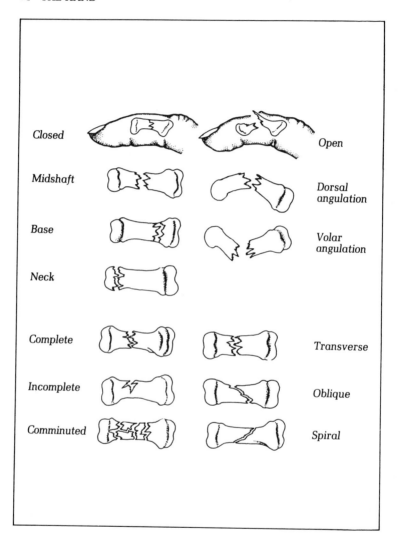

Figure 34
Fracture terminology

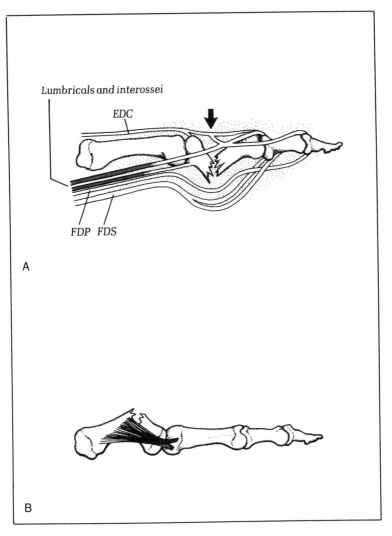

Figure 35

Deforming force acting on fracture site *(A)* The intrinsics flex the proximal fragment of the proximal phalanx; the intrinsic flexor and extensor with longitudinal pull cause further buckling at the fracture site *(B)* The intrinsic muscle cuses flexion deformity of metacarpal fracture.

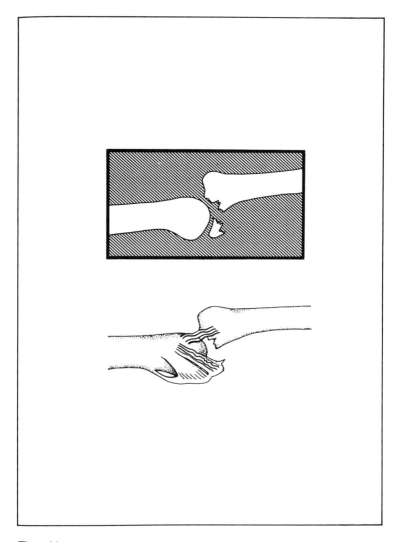

Figure 36
Unstable fracture-dislocation of PIP joint with volar fragment;
radiographic appearance above; ligament attachments, below

It is apparent from the following examples that a knowledge of the functional anatomy of the soft tissues related to the joints of the hand is essential to understanding these potentially disabling injuries. The radiographs can misleadingly suggest that a very simple fracture has occurred with only a small fragment of the bone involved. This fragment, however, is often the major attachment of a collateral ligament, the volar plate, or a tendon. This small fracture may render the joint grossly or potentially unstable. Since many of these articular fractures were actually dislocations at the time of injury, the x-ray film may not indicate the true degree of original displacement that occurred.

INTRA-ARTICULAR FRACTURES

Particular attention should be directed to intra-articular fractures around the PIP joint (Fig. 36). These often involve injuries to the volar plate and portions of the collateral ligaments. The early objective evidence of this may be seen radiographically as small, avulsed fragments of bone around the joint. When a volar triangular fracture fragment from the middle phalanx involves more than one quarter of the articular surface, dorsal dislocation of the middle phalanx *may* occur late because the volar plate and a significant portion of the collateral ligaments are attached to this small fragment. Because of this instability, these fractures often require surgical treatment. Early recognition and proper treatment depend on an awareness of the importance of these initial radiographic findings. Undertreatment is a common cause of disability.

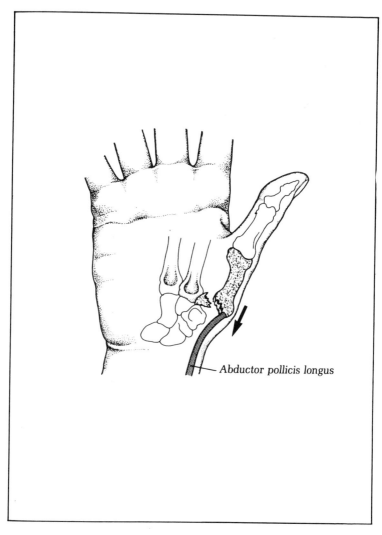

Abductor pollicis longus

Figure 37
Bennett's fracture

BENNETT'S FRACTURE

Bennett's fracture is an oblique intra-articular fracture from the ulnar base of the thumb metacarpal (Fig. 37). The palmar-ulnar portion of the metacarpal, which with its heavy ligamentous attachments normally stabilizes this joint, is separated from the larger distal fragment which is displaced by the pull of the APL.

FIFTH CMC FRACTURE-DISLOCATION

As in the thumb, an intra-articular fracture involving the palmar articular surface of the base of the fifth metacarpal may be unstable. This occurs as a result of the joint's relative mobility and the proximal pull of the ECU, which inserts onto the dorso-ulnar base of the fifth metacarpal.

BOXER'S FRACTURE

"Boxer's fracture" usually involves the acute angulation of the head of the metacarpal of the small finger into the palm, as the result of a blow on the distal-dorsal aspect of the closed fist. A loss of prominence of the metacarpal head is often seen on physical examination. The active motion of the small finger may be minimally disturbed on initial examination.

FRACTURE OF THE SCAPHOID

The bone most commonly fractured in the wrist is the scaphoid. There is tenderness on deep palpation in the snuff box area of the wrist just distal to the radial styloid

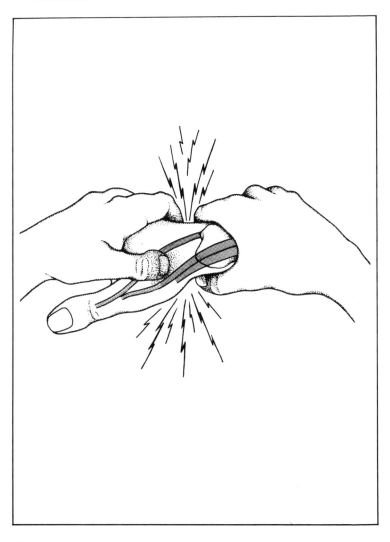

Figure 38
Fracture of scaphoid with tenderness on deep palpation in the
snuff box area

(Fig. 38). An oblique radiograph (scaphoid view) will usually best show the fracture. Frequently the initial radiograph will fail to show the fracture, whereas repeat views of the scaphoid taken 2 weeks later may show it after there has been resorption of bone at the fracture site. In all wrist injuries with snuff box tenderness, careful evaluation with adequate follow-up is required to make certain that these occult fractures are not overlooked.

Radionuclide imaging is an extremely effective means of confirming or ruling out the presence of a scaphoid fracture. The test can be performed as early as 24 hours after injury.

THE MCP JOINT DISLOCATION

The thumb may be subjected to significant hyperextension forces. The MCP volar plate may be disrupted at its metacarpal attachment with a hyperextension injury, and the joint may dislocate so that the proximal phalanx comes to lie dorsal to the metacarpal head which buttonholes between the intrinsic muscles and the FPL.

Similarly, the finger MCP joint (most commonly index or small) may dislocate, with the metacarpal head becoming entrapped between the flexor tendon ulnarly, the lumbrical musculotendinous unit radially, and the volar plate dorsally.

These dislocations can only be detected on true lateral radiographs and almost always require open reduction.

TORN ULNAR COLLATERAL LIGAMENT OF THE MCP JOINT OF THE THUMB

Acute radial deviation of the thumb at the MCP joint may disrupt the ulnar collateral ligament. It is commonly

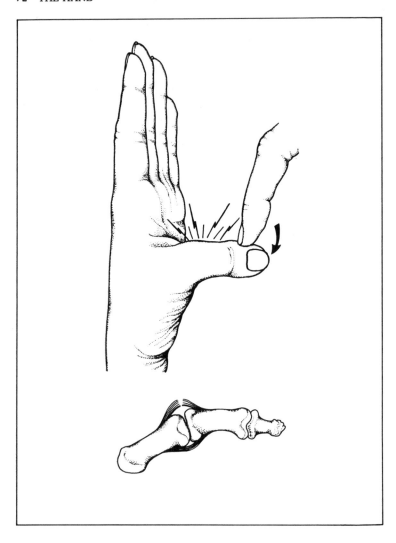

Figure 39
Rupture of ulnar collateral ligament of the MCP joint of the thumb

caused by falls while skiing, in which the thumb is forcefully radially deviated by the ski pole or strap when the hand hits the ground. It is important to compare the joint stability of the injured thumb with the patient's uninjured thumb. The lateral stress should be applied with the MCP joint in 15° to 20° of flexion and in full flexion. This test can be done clinically or under radiographic control. If the radial deviation of the thumb on stress testing with local wrist block anesthesia is 15° greater than that of the uninjured thumb, the collateral ligament is probably disrupted. Surgical repair is usually advisable (Fig. 39).

5

ACQUIRED DEFORMITIES

Deformities of the hand may be congenital or acquired. The acquired deformities may be associated with previous traumatic injuries to joints, tendons, or nerves, with progressively contracting fascia of the palm, or with arthritis. A discussion of some of the common deformities is presented.

MALLET FINGER

The mallet finger is a flexion posture or "droop" of the finger at the DIP joint area in which there is complete passive but incomplete active extension of the DIP joint (Fig. 40). The cause of the injury is usually a sudden blow to the tip of the extended finger. The insertion of the extensor tendon may be avulsed, or there may be an avulsion fracture of the distal phalanx with a dorsal piece of bone still attached to the extensor tendon. The PIP joint should always be examined to rule out co-existing injury. Anteroposterior and true lateral radiographs of the PIP and DIP joints are part of the examination. A laceration over the dorsum of the distal joint may sever the extensor tendon and result in a mallet finger deformity.

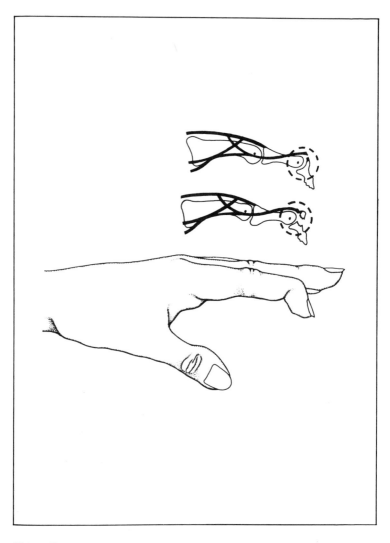

Figure 40
Mallet finger deformity (with or without fracture)

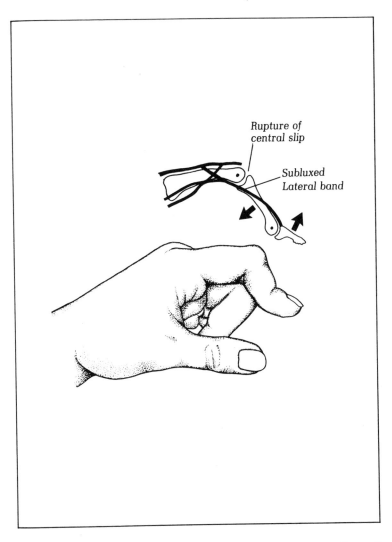

Rupture of
central slip

Subluxed
Lateral band

Figure 41
Boutonnière deformity

BOUTONNIÈRE DEFORMITY

In boutonnière deformity of the finger there is flexion of the PIP joint and hyperextension of the DIP joint (Fig. 41). It is the result of an injury or disease disrupting the extensor tendon insertion into the dorsal base of the middle phalanx. The fibers maintaining the position of the lateral bands progressively tear or stretch, allowing the lateral bands to slip volar to the axis of the PIP joint, with the result that they become flexors of the PIP. The deformity may not be present, however, immediately following the injury, but can develop over several days or weeks as the lateral bands drift progressively volarward.

SWAN-NECK DEFORMITY

This deformity of the finger is one in which the PIP joint is in hyperextension with the DIP joint in flexion (Fig. 42). It can be seen in a variety of conditions such as rheumatoid arthritis, certain types of spasticity, PIP joint volar plate injury, or old mallet finger deformity.

CLAW HAND

Claw hand deformity is manifest by flattening of the transverse metacarpal arch and longitudinal arches, with hyperextension of the MCP joints and flexion of the PIP and DIP joints (Figs. 28 and 43). The deformity is produced by an imbalance of the intrinsic and extrinsic muscles. The intrinsic muscles must be markedly weakened or paralyzed. The long extensor muscles hyperextend the MCP joint, and the long flexor muscles flex the PIP and DIP joints. Loss of intrinsic muscle function is

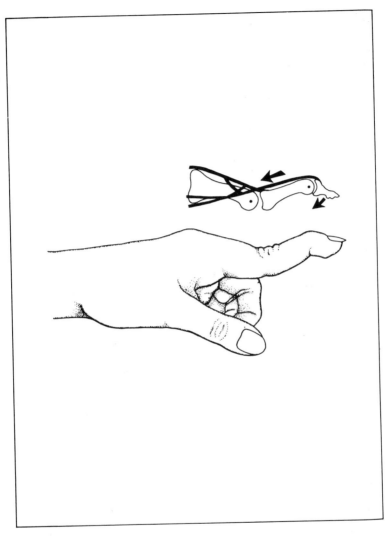

Figure 42
Swan-neck deformity

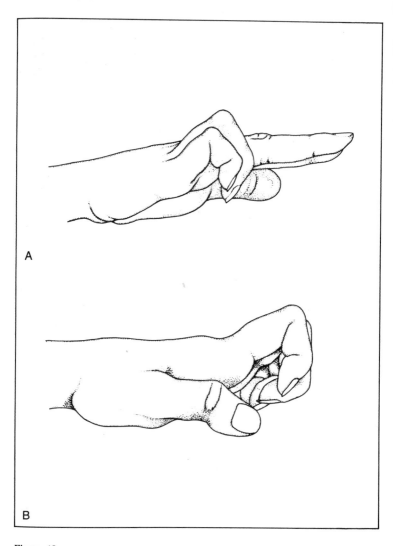

Figure 43
Claw hand deformity associated with *(A)* ulnar nerve palsy and
(B) combined median and ulnar nerve palsy

sometimes referred to as an "intrinsic minus hand." This deformity can be seen in such anomalies as ulnar nerve lesions, combined median and ulnar nerve lesions, brachial plexus injuries, spinal cord injuries, and Charcot-Marie-Tooth disease.

DUPUYTREN'S CONTRACTURE

Dupuytren's contracture is a contracture of the proliferated longitudinal bands of the palmar aponeurosis lying between the skin and flexor tendons in the distal palm and fingers (Fig. 44). The flexor tendons are not involved. It occurs most often in the ring and small fingers. It begins as a nodule and progresses to fibrous bands, with contracture of the fingers. It is usually not painful and is most often seen in older men. It is often familial.

RHEUMATOID ARTHRITIS

Rheumatoid arthritis in the hand usually starts with stiff, swollen, painful fingers. The MCP and PIP joints are the ones most frequently involved. Stiffness and pain are worse on arising in the morning. As the disease progresses, the digits often become deformed and the classic ulnar drift deformity of the fingers may develop (Fig. 45). Swan-neck and boutonnière deformities are common. Carpal tunnel syndrome, trigger finger, wrist tenosynovitis, painful flexor tenosynovitis, and rupture of tendons may be present.

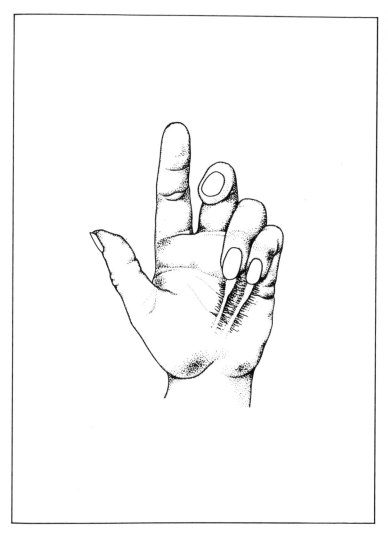

Figure 44
Dupuytren's contracture

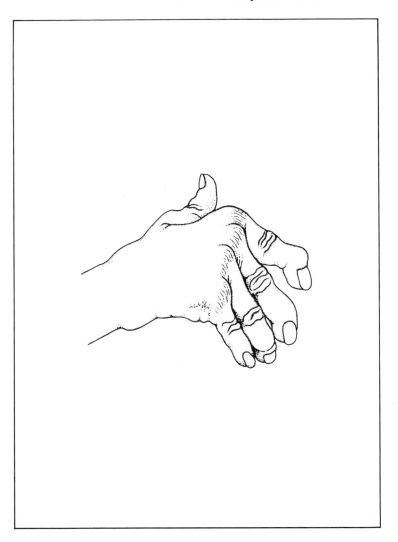

Figure 45
Rheumatoid arthritis of the hand with ulnar drift

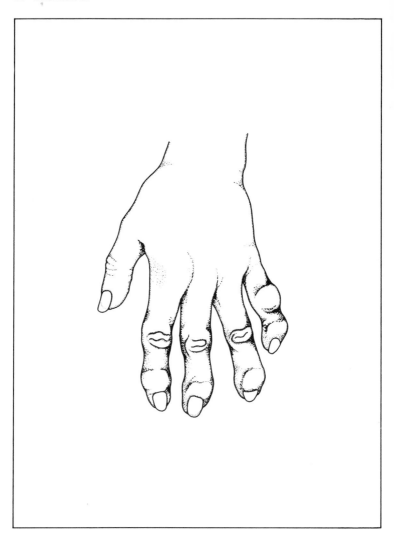

Figure 46
Degenerative arthritis of the hand

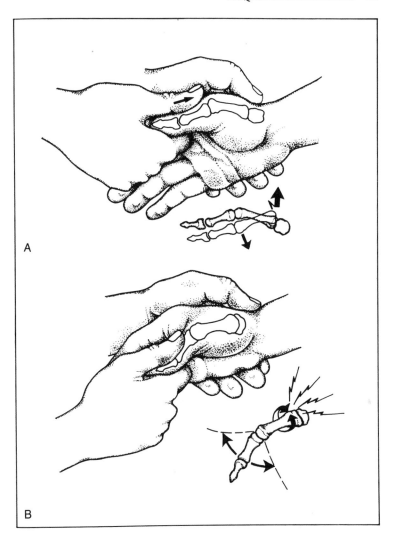

Figure 47
(A) Axial compression-adduction test *(B)* Axial compression and rotation test

DEGENERATIVE ARTHRITIS

In degenerative arthritis (osteoarthritis) of the hand, the distal joints develop marginal osteophytes known as Heberden's nodes (Fig. 46). Similar bony lesions, called Bouchard's nodes, may occur at the PIP joint. The MCP joints are seldom involved.

The CMC joint of the thumb is also a common site for degenerative arthritis in the hand. The axial compression-adduction test (Fig. 47) is done by manipulating the thumb with axial compression and gentle adduction. The instability and crepitus are appreciated with the examining thumb placed on the joint and base of metacarpal. This is usually painful for the patient with joint involvement. The axial compression and rotation (Fig. 47) are often painful when the proximal phalanx is used as a lever arm for a grinding maneuver of the thumb CMC joint.

DEQUERVAIN'S TENOSYNOVITIS

A nonspecific tenosynovitis of the APL and EPB tendons in the first dorsal wrist compartment is known as deQuervain's disorder. Tenderness and crepitation may be present over the radial styloid. Finkelstein's test may be positive (Fig. 48). It is performed by having the patient grasp the thumb with the fingers (thumb in palm) and ulnar deviate the wrist. If this causes pain the test is positive.

It is important to differentiate between deQuervain's tenosynovitis and CMC joint arthrosis of the thumb. To do this, tenderness and pain must be accurately localized between this first extensor compartment and the CMC joint of the thumb. Radiographs should be taken if there is uncertainty.

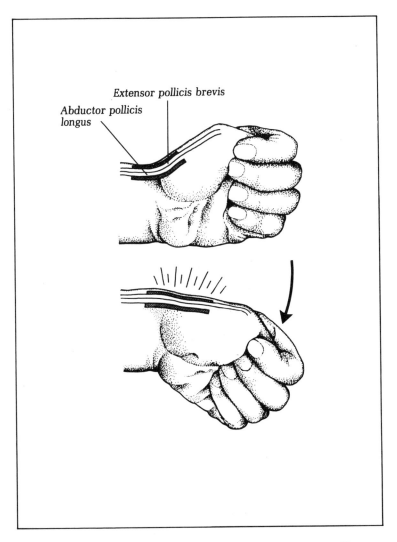

Figure 48
Finkelstein's test for deQuervain's disease

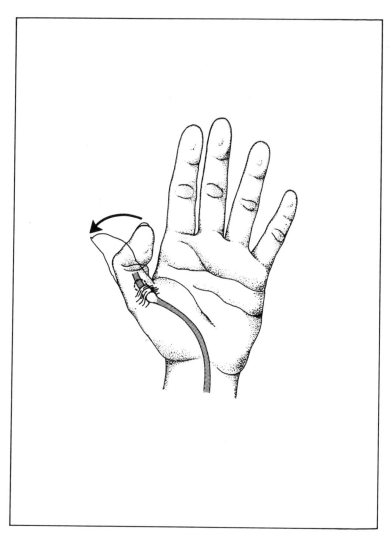

Figure 49
Trigger thumb

TRIGGER THUMB AND TRIGGER FINGER

Stenosing tenosynovitis can occur in the thumb or any finger, but it most commonly occurs in the ring or middle fingers. Inflammation at the MCP joint pulley causes a discrepancy between the size of the tendon and pulley. The tendon may become thickened just proximal to the pulley. This discrepancy in size may cause a snapping or locking phenomenon, holding the thumb or finger flexed or extended (Fig. 49). Palpation of the flexor tendon over the MCP joint can be painful.

CARPAL TUNNEL SYNDROME

The carpal tunnel syndrome is a median nerve compression neuropathy at the wrist where the nerve passes beneath the transverse carpal ligament (Fig. 50). Patients complain of their hands "going to sleep" and are frequently awakened at night with numbness, pain, and tingling in the thumb, index, long, and ring fingers. The small finger is not usually involved. Patients may complain of referred pain in the forearm and even as high as the shoulder. They notice these symptoms when driving a car or during other sustained activities. The entity is more common in women than men. The dominant hand is more often involved but symptoms can be bilateral. The carpal tunnel syndrome may be associated with rheumatoid arthritis or following a Colles' fracture. It can also be seen in a variety of medical conditions such as pregnancy, diabetes mellitus, and thyroid disease. However, most patients with the carpal tunnel syndrome have no apparent associated systemic disease.

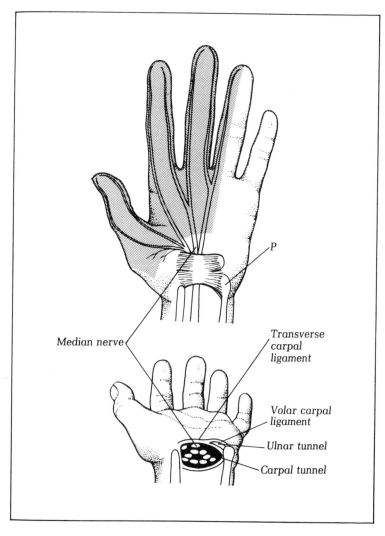

Figure 50
Carpal tunnel syndrome (median nerve compression syndrome)

The hand will most often look normal; however, in long-standing cases there may be atrophy of the median innervated thenar muscles (Fig. 51).

Tapping over the median nerve at the wrist crease may produce paresthesias in the hand (Tinel's sign) (Fig. 52). The wrist flexion test (Phalen's test) (Fig. 53) is done by resting the elbows on a table and allowing the wrists to fall into complete volar flexion for 1 minute. If the patient has carpal tunnel syndrome, this position may produce paresthesias in the hand. If the patient is unable to flex the wrist as a result of pain or limited motion, direct compression of the median nerve can be accomplished by applying pressure with the thumb in the interval between the PL and FCR tendons at the level of the distal wrist flexion crease for 1 to 2 minutes duration. The development of discomfort or paresthesias in the distribution of the median nerve or an asymmetry in onset of symptoms when compared with the opposite wrist suggests possible carpal tunnel syndrome.

CUBITAL TUNNEL SYNDROME

Numbness or paresthesias in the ring and small fingers of the hand suggests the possibility of entrapment neuropathy of the ulnar nerve. The ulnar nerve is susceptible to compression in the cubital tunnel at the elbow and Guyon's canal at the wrist. The cubital tunnel is the fibro-osseous canal, which stabilizes the ulnar nerve as it passes behind the medial epicondyle of the humerus. There are multiple causes for injury to the ulnar nerve at this location including hypermobility or subluxation of the nerve from the cubital tunnel, and changes in the anatomic alignment of the elbow. Compression injury of the ulnar nerve within the cubital tunnel can be identified

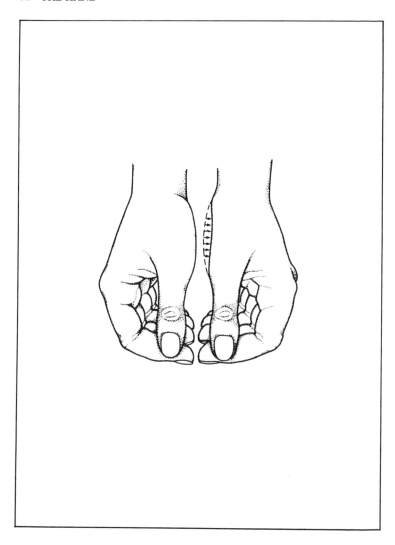

Figure 51
Atrophy of the thenar muscle

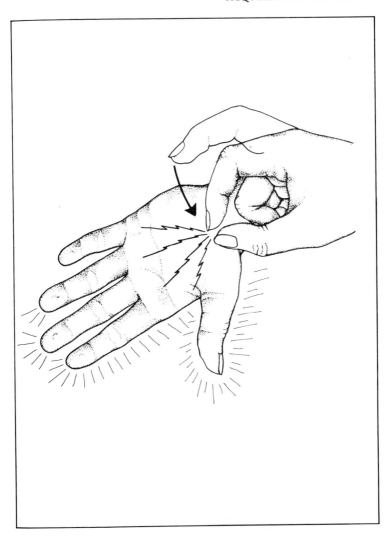

Figure 52
Tinel's sign

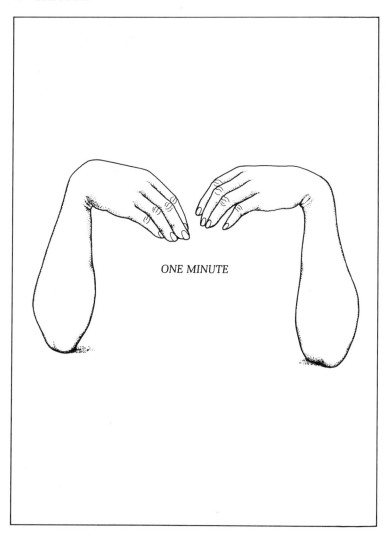

ONE MINUTE

Figure 53
Phalen's sign (wrist flexion test)

by a painful Tinel's sign and the onset of paresthesias in the ring and small fingers with elbow flexion under 2 minutes. With entrapment of the ulnar nerve at the cubital tunnel, there may be numbness over the dorso-ulnar aspect of the hand in addition to paresthesias in the ring and small fingers. In more severe cases of cubital tunnel syndrome, there will be decreased 2PD in the sensory distribution of the ulnar nerve as well as muscle weakness and/or wasting of the intrinsic muscles innervated by the ulnar nerve. Clinical findings include a positive Froment's test, wasting of the first dorsal interosseous muscle, inability to cross the index and middle fingers, and clawing of the ring and small fingers.

Entrapment of the ulnar nerve at the wrist may demonstrate a positive Tinel's sign on percussion over the ulnar nerve at Guyon's canal and a positive Phalen's test with paresthesias in the ring and small fingers. It will not demonstrate loss of sensation over the dorso-ulnar aspect of the hand. Depending on the site and severity of compression, there may be diminished 2PD and/or ulnar intrinsic muscle weakness.

LATERAL EPICONDYLITIS

Although sometimes referred to as tennis elbow, this condition most commonly develops in individuals who perform repetitive manual labor. The injury appears to involve a detachment of the origin of the ECRB from the lateral epicondyle. The injury is aggravated by lifting with the forearm in a position of pronation and the wrist held in extension. Examination demonstrates point tenderness over the lateral epicondyle. The patient's pain can be reproduced by having the patient extend the wrist against resistance with the elbow held in extension and the forearm in pronation.

6

CONGENITAL ANOMALIES

Congenital defects are often encountered in the examination of the hand. These defects should be recorded in an accurate and complete manner. In the past, the use of various Greek and Latin names to describe common deficiencies has only served to confuse many clinicians. A classification should be used that groups cases according to the parts that have been affected primarily by certain embryologic failures.

The various clinical pictures of limb deficiencies are felt to represent varying degrees of destruction within the ectomesenchymal mass that develops on the lateral body wall of the developing embryo. The limb bud is first noted at the fourth week after gestation. These buds grow and differentiate rapidly in a proximodistal sequence during the following four weeks. Any factor, environmental or otherwise, that disrupts the sequential differentiation during this period will produce a defect in the limb compatible with the timing of the insult.

Congenital defects should be classified in the following categories as outlined by the American Society for Surgery of the Hand and the International Federation of Societies for Surgery of the Hand:

1. Failure of formation of parts (arrest of development).
2. Failure of differentiation (separation) of parts.
3. Duplication.
4. Overgrowth (gigantism).
5. Undergrowth (hypoplasia).
6. Congenital constriction band syndrome.
7. Generalized skeletal abnormalities.

FAILURE OF FORMATION OF PARTS

The category of failure of formation of parts is that group of congenital deficiencies noted by failure or arrest of formation of the limb either complete or partial. This category is divided into two types: transverse and longitudinal.

Transverse deficiencies

Transverse deficiencies represent the so-called congenital amputations ranging from aphalangia (absence of the fingers) to amelia (absence of the extremity). The stumps are usually well-padded and may show rudimentary digits or dimpling. One of the most common defects in the group is the short below elbow amputation. This would be classified as a transverse (T), left or right (L-R), forearm (FO), upper one third deficiency.

Longitudinal deficiencies

Longitudinal deficiencies include all other limb deficiencies in this category. In identifying longitudinal deficiencies, all completely or partially absent bones are named.

The deficiencies in the group reflect the separation of the pre-axial (radial) and post-axial (ulnar) divisions in the limb and include longitudinal failure of formation of the entire limb segment (phocomelias) of either radial, central, or ulnar components of the limb.

An example of a segmental failure would be the phocomelia (hand attached to the trunk). This would be classified: longitudinal (L), left or right (L-R), humerus (Hu), radius (Ra), ulna (Ul).

The absence of parts of the radial (pre-axial) side of the limb may vary from deficient thenar muscles to a short floating thumb, and from deficient carpals, metacarpals, and radius to the classified so-called radial club hand. The classification of longitudinal, right, radius, proximal one third, carpal partial, first ray, would be a deficiency with a partial absence of the radius and carpal bones with no thumb on the right.

Central deficiencies include deficiencies of the middle three digits: index, long, and ring, and sometimes the carpal bones. The middle digit may be missing in the so-called lobster claw hand.

In ulnar deficiencies, the small or ring finger may be missing and can be associated with partial or complete absence of the ulna and carpal bones. These are classified in a like manner.

FAILURE OF DIFFERENTIATION (SEPARATION) OF PARTS

Failure of differentiation is that category in which the basic units have developed but the final form is not completed. The homogenous anlage divides into separate tissues of skeletal, dermomyofascial, or neurovascular elements found in normal limbs, but fails to differentiate completely or to separate. An example in the forearm would be a synostosis (fusion of bones which are normally separated) of the proximal radius and ulna. In the wrist, fusion of carpal bones is frequently seen as well as fusion of two or more metacarpals. Synphalangism is end-to-end fusion of the proximal interphalangeal joints. Syndactyly is by far the most common deformity seen in this category. The failure of differentiation can vary from simple skin bridging to fusion of parts.

Contractures secondary to failure of differentiation of muscle, ligaments, and capsular structure are frequently seen. They vary from simple trigger thumb to flexion contractures of the small finger (camptodactyly) to the severe arthrogryposis of the hand.

Lateral deviation or displacement due to asymmetrical abnormalities of the digits (clinodactyly) also occurs.

DUPLICATION

Duplication of parts probably occurs as a result of a particular insult to the limb bud and ectodermal cap at a very early stage of their development so that splitting of the original embryonic part occurs. These defects may range from polydactyly (too many digits) to twinning or mirror hand (duplication of the digits present). They are classified according to the parts or tissues duplicated. Polydactyly is the most common deformity seen in this group. It can be either radial (duplication of the thumb, partial or complete), central (middle three fingers) or ulnar (small finger duplication, partial or complete). The thumb and small finger duplications are seen more frequently.

OVERGROWTH (GIGANTISM)

In this category, there can be overgrowth of the entire limb or a single part. Some cases appear to be due to skeletal overgrowth with normal-appearing soft tissue. Others show excess fat, lymphatic, and fibrous tissue; neurofibromata, lymphangiomata, or angiomata may be present in these cases. A frequently seen deformity in this category is gigantism of the digit and there can be an accompanying syndactyly. This would be classified as an overgrowth (gigantism) of the digit with syndactyly as a secondary condition.

UNDERGROWTH (HYPOPLASIA)

Undergrowth or hypoplasia denotes defective or incomplete development of the parts. This may be manifested in the entire extremity or its divisions. Hypoplasia may involve any of the following systems: skin and nails, musculotendinous, neurovascular, or the extremity (arm, forearm, hand). An abnormally short, completely formed metacarpal would be brachymetacarpia. Brachyphalangia refers to abnormally short middle phalanges.

CONGENITAL CONSTRICTION BAND SYNDROME

This abnormality involves a circumferential constriction of soft tissues of the extremity. Whether this is a developmental defect or mechanical constriction secondary to aminiotic bands remains uncertain. Compromise in the development of the soft tissues distal to the site of constriction may be associated with soft tissue fusion of the distal parts, or may produce actual amputation. Those cases producing vascular compromise require surgery to maintain the viability of the affected part.

GENERALIZED SKELETAL ABNORMALITIES (MADELUNG'S DEFORMITY)

This congenital anomaly involves a hypoplasia of the distal ulna and ulnar aspect of the distal radius. It is more common in females than males and is typically bilateral. The deformity may not become detectable until the child reaches adolescence. A similar deformity can sometimes be produced by infection or trauma.

7

TUMORS

The most common soft tissue mass of the hand is a ganglion (Fig. 54). It has a well-defined, smooth surface and is a firm cystic lesion that is fixed to the deep tissues. It may develop over the volar or dorsal area of the wrist, originating from the wrist capsule. Those in the palm near the digital palmar skin crease arise from the flexor tendon sheath and may or may not be painful.

A mucous cyst is a cystic lesion (actually a ganglion) over the dorsum of the finger near the distal joint and fingernail (Fig. 55). It is associated with degenerative arthritis of the DIP joint of the finger and arises from the joint. It may have thin walls and there may be associated grooving of the fingernail distal to the cyst. Should a mucous cyst rupture and become infected, a septic joint may result.

Other soft tissue tumors of the hand that may present as a mass are giant cell tumors of tendon sheath, pigmented villonodular synovitis, and inclusion cysts.

Malignant tumors of the soft tissue and bone are rare in the hand. However, skin cancers (basal cell and squamous cell) on the dorsum of the hand are seen in the elderly. Malignant melanoma does occur in the hand and may be subungual.

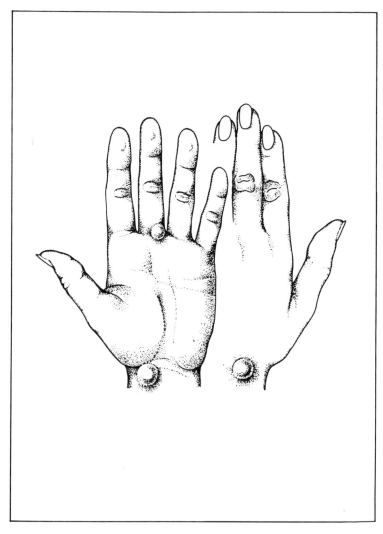

Figure 54
Ganglion of the hand

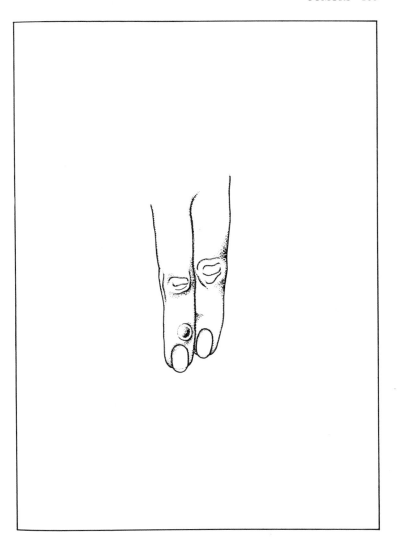

Figure 55
Mucous cyst

Primary bone tumors of the hand usually present as swelling and/or pain in the area of the hand involved. The tumor is located radiographically and the diagnosis is established by biopsy of the tumor. The most common bone tumor of the hand is an enchondroma. It is often first discovered when a fracture occurs through the lesion.

8

INFECTION

PARONYCHIA

A paronychia is an infection of the soft tissue around the fingernail that usually begins as a "hangnail" and that is usually caused by a staphylococcus infection (Fig. 56A). It spreads around the nail eponychium, thus the term "run around." It is red, swollen, and very painful, with purulent drainage around the margin of the nail.

FELON

A felon is a deep infection of the pulp space of the distal segment of the finger (Fig. 56B). The distal segment is swollen, red, and extremely painful. Drainage is usually required. It is usually caused by a staphylococcus infection and can involve the distal phalanx with osteomyelitis.

PURULENT TENOSYNOVITIS

Infection of the tendon sheath of the digit presents as a swollen, slightly flexed finger with tenderness over the

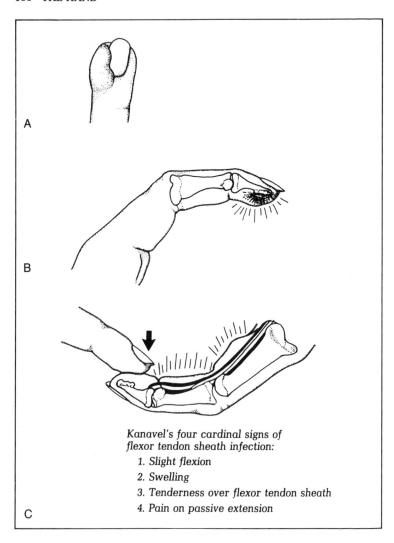

Kanavel's four cardinal signs of
flexor tendon sheath infection:

    1. Slight flexion

    2. Swelling

    3. Tenderness over flexor tendon sheath

    4. Pain on passive extension

Figure 56
(A) Paronychia *(B)* Felon *(C)* Flexor tendon sheath infection

flexor tendon sheath and increased pain on passive extension of the digit (Fig. 56C). These findings constitute Kanavel's four cardinal signs of a purulent tendon sheath infection.

If the tendon sheath of the small finger or thumb is involved primarily, the infection may spread to the wrist area where the sheaths communicate and the classic "horseshoe" infection may develop (Fig. 57). The sheath of the index, long, and ring fingers extends to the palm but not to the wrist. Streptococcus and staphylococcus are the most frequent infecting organisms.

These are serious infections which may extend along the flexor tendon sheath, and prompt treatment is most important.

SPACE INFECTIONS

Thenar space and mid-palm infections are not common. When they do occur the dorsum may be more swollen than the palm of the hand. This should not mislead the examiner. The usual findings of redness, tenderness, and perhaps fluctuance help to define the abscess.

The thenar space is a potential space anterior to the adductor muscle (Fig. 58). Its ulnar border is separated from the mid-palm space by a fascia arising from the metacarpal of the long finger and attaching to the palmar fascia.

The mid-palm space is the potential space anterior to the interosseous muscles and posterior to the flexor tendons of the long, ring, and small fingers (Fig. 59).

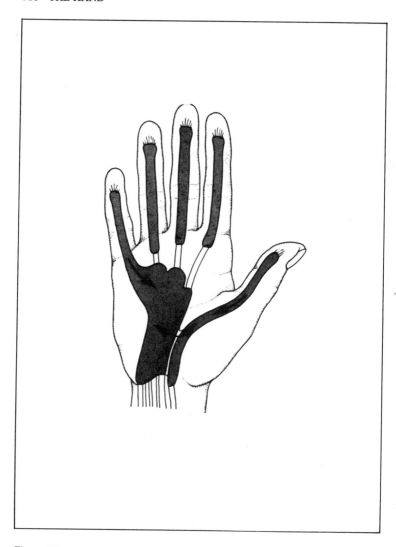

Figure 57
Tendon sheaths of the flexor tendon

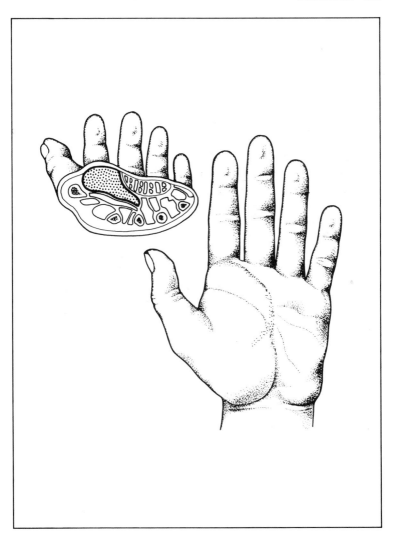

Figure 58
Thenar space infection of the hand

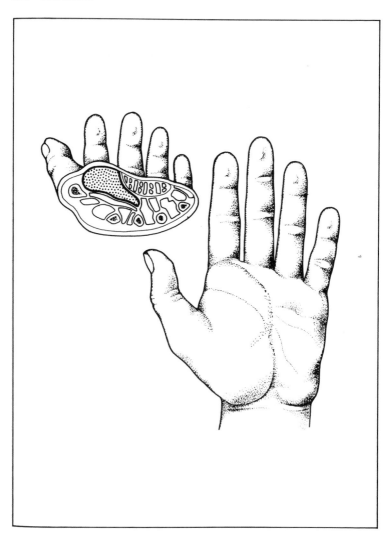

Figure 59
Mid-palm space infection of the hand

HUMAN BITE INFECTIONS

Human bites are commonly seen over the dorsum of the MCP joints. These usually occur when the joint area strikes a tooth in a fight. The important point is that the wound may appear benign initially, but is usually inoculated with a potent mixture of bacterial flora. This is a serious injury requiring prompt treatment.

APPENDIX 1

KEY TO ABBREVIATIONS USED IN THE TEXT

ADM	Abductor digiti minimi
AdP	Adductor pollicis
APB	Abductor pollicis brevis
APL	Abductor pollicis longus
CMC	Carpometacarpal
DIP	Distal interphalangeal
ECRB	Extensor carpi radialis brevis
ECRL	Extensor carpi radialis longus
ECU	Extensor carpi ulnaris
EDC	Extensor digitorum communis
EDM	Extensor digiti minimi
EIP	Extensor indicis proprius
EPB	Extensor pollicis brevis
EPL	Extensor pollicis longus
FCR	Flexor carpi radialis
FCU	Flexor carpi ulnaris
FDM	Flexor digiti minimi
FDP	Flexor digitorum profundus
FDS	Flexor digitorum superficialis
FPB	Flexor pollicis brevis
FPL	Flexor pollicis longus
I	Index finger
IP	Interphalangeal
M	Middle finger

MCP	Metacarpophalangeal
ODM	Opponens digiti minimi
OP	Opponens pollicis
PIP	Proximal interphalangeal
PL	Palmaris longus
R	Ring finger
S	Small finger

APPENDIX 2

ANATOMY—SUMMARY

Joint Control	Prime* Muscle	Nerve	Fig. No.†	Comments
Wrist				
Flexion	FCR PL FCU	Median Median Ulnar		Absence—weak wrist flexion present by FDS, FDP
Extension	ECRL ECRB	Radial	8, 10, 13	Absence—"wrist drop"
Radial deviation	ECRL FCR	Radial Median		
Ulnar deviation	ECU FCU	Radial Ulnar		
Finger MCP				
Flexion	Interosseous Lumbrical	Ulnar Median I. & M.; Ulnar R. & S.	43	Absence—claw hand
Extension	EDC EIP	Radial	8, 12, 32	Absence—MCP extensor lag
Abduction	Dorsal Interosseous	Ulnar	16,17	
Adduction	Volar Interosseous	Ulnar		

Action	Muscles	Nerve	No.	Comments
Finger PIP Flexion	FDS	Median	7	Must block FDP to detect clinical absence
Extension	Interosseous, Lumbrical, EDC, EIP, EDM	Ulnar, Median & Ulnar, Radial	43	Intrinsic independent of MCP position: extrinsic only if MCP joint flexed or at 0° (i.e., not hyperextended)
Finger DIP Flexion	FDP	Median, I. & M.; Ulnar R. & S.	6	
Extension	None	—		Strong DIP extension contingent upon active PIP extension control
Thumb CMC Flexion-adduction	AdP, Ulnar ½ FPB, 1st dorsal interosseous, FPL	Ulnar, Ulnar or Median, Median	15	
Extension-abduction	EPL, EPB, APL, APB	Radial, Radial, Median	9,11	

Joint Control	Prime* Muscle	Nerve	Fig. No.†	Comments
Opposition (Pronation)	APB Radial ½ FPB OP	Median	3B, 14	A composite motion
Supination	EPL	Radial		
Thumb MCP Flexion	FPL thenar intrinsic muscles (except OP)	Median Median Ulnar		
Extension	EPB	Radial	9	
Thumb IP Flexion	FPL	Median	5	
Extension	EPL	Radial	11	Weak IP extension also by intrinsics

(*achieves a given function but does not imply 'the strongest' acting across that joint)
(†in addition to Figs. 19, 20, 22)

APPENDIX 3

CLINICAL ASSESSMENT RECOMMENDATIONS

SENSIBILITY

Two-point discrimination, with the use of a blunt instrument, applied in a longitudinal axis of the digit (see Fig. 24). Pressure applied that does not blanch skin.

Ratings

1. Normal, less than 6 mm.
2. Fair, 6 to 10 mm.
3. Poor, 11 to 15 mm.
4. Protective, one point perceived.
5. Anesthetic, no point perceived.

STRENGTH

Grip strength

Use a squeeze (grip) dynamometer and make three successive determinations. The correct position for recording grip strength is with the arm comfortably at the patient's side, the elbow flexed at 90°, and the forearm and hand resting unsupported. Record and calculate post-treatment percentage relative to pre-treatment value as well as to value from the contralateral hand. **Note**: This is *not* a percentage of physical impairment or improvement but merely an indicator of improving or worsening condition.

Pinch strength

Use a pinch dynamometer. Key pinch is the thumb tip to radial aspect of middle phalanx of the index finger and is the most universal and preferred value. Record three successive efforts and calculate percentage relative to pre-treatment as well as contralateral hand values. Tip pinch value (reverse key pinch —index tip to ulnar tip of thumb) will be less powerful than key pinch. Same recordings as for key pinch. **Note**: This is *not* a percentage of physical impairment or improvement but merely an indicator of improving or worsening condition.

MOTION

Total passive motion (TPM)

Sum of angles formed by MCP, PIP, and DIP joints in maximum passive flexion minus the sum of angles of deficit from complete extension at each of these three joints: (MCP + PIP + DIP) − (MCP + PIP + DIP) = total flexion − total extensor lag TPM.

Total active motion (TAM)

Sum of angles formed by MCP, PIP, and DIP joints in maximum active flexion, i.e., fist position, minus total extension deficity at the MCP, PIP, and DIP joints with active finger extension. Significant hyperextension at any joint, particularly the PIP and DIP joints, is recorded as a deficit in extension and is included in the total extension deficit. Hyperextension must be considered an abnormal value in swan-neck, (PIP) and boutonnière deformities (DIP). Comparison of pre- and post-treatment TAM values will be significant; however, comparison as a percentage of normal value is invalid.

TAM is a term applied to one finger, and is analagous to TPM in calculation except that only active motion is recorded, not passive.

1. Sum of active MCP flexion + active PIP flexion + active DIP flexion.
2. Minus sum of incomplete active extension (if any is present).

It is of critical importance to emphasize that this system of measuring and recording joint motions is used in the following situations:

1. For a single digit
2. To indicate the total motion of that digit in degrees
3. To compare this to subsequent measurements of that same digit or the corresponding normal digit of the opposite hand in the same patient to determine if the patient is gaining or losing motion

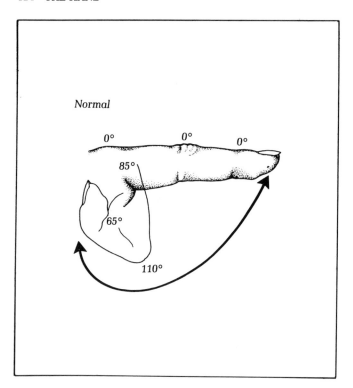

Normal

Active	Flexion	Extension Lack
MCP	85°	0°
PIP	110°	0°
DIP	65°	0°
Totals	260°	0°

Total Active Motion (TAM)
260° − 0° = 260°

Figure 60

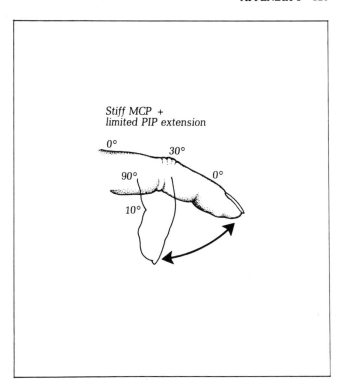

*Stiff MCP +
limited PIP extension*

Stiff MCP + Limited PIP Extension

Active	Flexion	Extension Lack
MCP	0°	0°
PIP	90°	30°
DIP	10°	0°
Totals	100°	30°

Total Active Motion (TAM)
100° − 30° = 70°

Figure 61

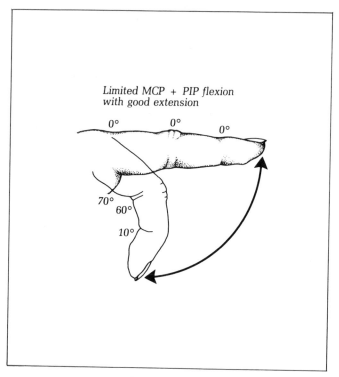

Limited MCP + PIP flexion
with good extension

Limited MCP + PIP Flexion with Good Extension

Active	Flexion	Extension Lack
MCP	70°	0°
PIP	60°	0°
DIP	10°	0°
Totals	140°	0°

Total Active Motion (TAM)
140° − 0° = 140°

Figure 62

It is not intended for the following:

1. To calculate a percentage of "functional improvement or loss"
2. To calculate a "percentage of impairment"

Note that some finger joints are more important than others in digital function. Furthermore, note that "function and impairment" involve many other factors as well, such as sensation.

VASCULAR STATUS

Patients who have vascular repair are evaluated in the following manner (not acutely, but late):

1. Examine for tissue survival.
2. Objective evidence of patent vessels by Allen test and for ultrasonic pulse detector.
3. Revascularized part examined in resting and post-exercise state by one of several methods:
   a. presence of capillary filling.
   b. physiologic testing such as ultrasonic pulse detector, skin temperatures, etc.

   When possible, comparison with evaluation before and after 3-minute tourniquet ischemia.
4. Evaluation regarding cold tolerance of the part.

Ratings

1. Failure, no survival.
2. Poor, tissue survival.
3. Fair, objective evidence of patent vessels.
4. Good, function not limited by circulation.
5. Excellent, no cold intolerance.

SUGGESTED READINGS

American Society for Surgery of the Hand: The Hand: Primary Care of Common Problems. 2nd. Ed. Churchill Livingstone, New York, 1990

Ariyan S: The Hand Book. 2nd. Ed. Williams & Wilkins, Baltimore, 1983

Beasley RW: Hand Injuries. WB Saunders, Philadelphia, 1981

Boswick JA, Jr: Current Concepts in Hand Surgery. Lea & Febiger, Philadelphia, 1983

Boswick JA, Jr: Complications in Hand Surgery. WB Saunders, Philadelphia, 1986

Boyes JH: Bunnell's Surgery of the Hand. 5th. Ed. JB Lippincott, Philadelphia, 1970

Buck-Gramcko D, Hoffman R, Neumann R: Hand Trauma. A Practical Guide. Thieme, New York, 1986

Burton RI: The hand. p. 273. In. Evarts MC (ed): Surgery of the Musculoskeletal System. 2nd. Ed. Churchill Livingstone, New York, 1990

Cailliet R: Hand Pain and Impairment. 3rd. Ed. FA Davis, Philadelphia, 1982

Carter PR: Common Hand Injuries and Infections: A Practical Approach to Early Treatment. WB Saunders, Philadelphia, 1983

Chase RA: Atlas of Hand Surgery. Vol. 1. WB Saunders, Philadelphia, 1973

Chase RA: Atlas of Hand Surgery. Vol. 2. WB Saunders, Philadelphia, 1983

Conolly WB: Color Atlas of Hand Conditions. Yearbook Medical Publishers, Chicago, 1980

Conolly WB, Kilgore ES, Jr: Hand Injuries and Infections, Yearbook Medical Publishers, Chicago, 1979

Flatt AE: The Care of Minor Hand Injuries. 3rd. Ed. CV Mosby, St. Louis, 1972

Flatt AE: Care of the Arthritic Hand. 4th. Ed. CV Mosby, St. Louis, 1983

Flynn JE: Hand Surgery. 3rd. Ed. Williams & Wilkins, Baltimore, 1982

Green DP: Operative Hand Surgery. 2nd. Ed. Churchill Livingstone, New York, 1988

Hunter JM, Schneider LH, Mackin EJ, Callahan AD: Rehabilitation of the Hand. 2nd. Ed. CV Mosby, St. Louis, 1984

Kilgore ES, Jr, Graham WP III: The Hand: Surgical and Nonsurgical Management. Lea & Febiger, Philadelphia, 1977

Lamb DW, Hooper G: Hand Conditions. Churchill Livingstone, Edinburgh, 1984

Lamb DW, Hooper G, Kuczynski MB: The Practice of Hand Surgery. 2nd. Ed. Blackwell Scientific, Boston, 1988

Lampe EW: Surgical anatomy of the hand. CIBA Clin Symp 40(3):1, 1988

Lister G: The Hand: Diagnosis and Indications. 2nd Ed. Churchill Livingstone, Edinburgh, 1984

Littler JW: The Hand and Upper Extremity. Vol. VI. In Converse JM (ed): Reconstructive Plastic Surgery. 2nd. Ed. WB Saunders, Philadelphia, 1977

Lucas GL: Examination of the Hand. Charles C Thomas, Springfield, IL, 1972

Macnicol MF, Lamb DW: Basic Care of the Injured Hand. Churchill Livingstone, Edinburgh, 1984

Mann RJ: Infections of the Hand. Lea & Febiger, Philadelphia, 1988

Milford L: The Hand. 3rd. Ed. CV Mosby, St. Louis, 1988

Newmeyer WL: Primary Care of Hand Injuries. Lea & Febiger, Philadelphia, 1979

Omer GE, Jr, Spinner M: Management of Peripheral Nerve Problems. WB Saunders, Philadelphia, 1980

Sandzen SC, Jr: Atlas of Wrist and Hand Fractures. PSG Publishing, Littleton, MA, 1979

Sandzen SC, Jr: Atlas of Acute Hand Injuries. McGraw-Hill, New York, 1980

Schamber D: Simply Performed Tests of the Hand. Vantage Press, New York, 1984

Semple C: The Primary Management of Hand Injuries. Yearbook Medical Publishers, Chicago, 1979

Spinner M: Injuries to the Major Branches of Peripheral Nerves of the Forearm. 2nd. Ed. WB Saunders, Philadelphia, 1978

Spinner M: Kaplan's Functional and Surgical Anatomy of the Hand. 3rd. Ed. JB Lippincott, Philadelphia, 1984

Strickland JW, Steichen JB: Difficult Problems in Hand Surgery. CV Mosby, St. Louis, 1982

Tubiana R, Thomine JM, Mackin E: Examination of the Hand and Upper Limb. WB Saunders, Philadelphia, 1984

Weckesser EC: Treatment of Hand Injuries: Preservation and Restoration of Function. Yearbook Medical Publishers, Chicago, 1974

Weeks PM, Wray RC: Management of Acute Hand Injuries. CV Mosby, St. Louis, 1978

Wolfert FG: Acute Hand Injuries —A Multispecialty Approach. Little Brown, Boston, 1980

Wynn-Parry CB: Rehabilitation of the Hand. 4th. Ed. Butterworth, Woburn, MA, 1981

INDEX

Page numbers followed by f indicate figures.